What people are saying about

You Are a Frequency

This book offers the reader a window into a variety of spiritual principles highlighted within the Esoteric Philosophy. With remarkable clarity, the author provides insightful understanding as to how these spiritual precepts are foundational to an emerging new paradigm related to health and wellness. It accents the notion that underlying the physical form is an energy body that has a vibrational influence on one's health and psychological well-being. *You Are a Frequency* is a must-read for anyone ready to explore the next step in their understanding of the energies underlying and influencing our individual lives, as well as humanity as a whole.

William Meader, author of *Shine Forth: The Soul's Magical Destiny*, Portland, Oregon, USA

This book offers the reader an in-depth understanding of the relationships and the energies of the Soul and the tripod vehicle of the mental, emotional and physical bodies. Debbie gives us clarity on how we can manifest well-being by working on our subtler bodies. We can take control of our lives by understanding how our thoughts and emotions have an impact on our health, and by integrating these bodies with the Soul, we can reach that wholeness. We are truly all a frequency which is within our power to change as we evolve through the Path of the Soul.

Astra Ferro, author of *Stepping Stones on the Spiritual Path, The Journey of the Soul through the Seven Major Chakras* and *Understanding the Soul's Journey through the L*____ ___ __

T0002065

A new paradigm of healthcare is long overdue. This book goes some way towards setting out why that is so and suggesting ways forward which are born out of who we are. In conventional healthcare, the GP is, invariably, the authority, leaving patients feeling powerless and unable to contribute to their own treatment. Debbie Sellwood skilfully brings together a number of important health and healing modalities which, together, represent a more sensitive and intelligent approach to healthcare, addressing the whole person rather than the physical body alone. She adopts a holistic view which explores the body's energy network and the profound roles of the mental and emotional bodies, and their impact on the physical. As the book unfolds, we begin to realize that we are far from powerless and that we can develop mental and emotional attitudes which are conducive to good health. For instance, when we insist on repeatedly re-living challenging circumstances, or suppress unfulfilled desires and emotions, we can so easily create dis-ease.

Drawing on wisdom and studies, both ancient and modern, and comparatively new sciences such as epigenetics, Debbie traces a path which is at once enlightening and uplifting. The implicit becomes explicit when, for instance, she devotes an entire chapter to exploring the possible reasons and purpose of illness. In Chapter 10 she looks at solutions for wellbeing and a way forward. Debbie envisions a future healthcare system awake to the circulation of life-force energy throughout the subtle bodies, meridian and chakra systems, leading to good health. Who among us does not desire good health and wellbeing? This book does what it says on the label and shows how our personal vibration influences health, wellness and development. Undoubtedly, it will help you to reflect on your own attitudes and ways of being.

Elizabeth Medler, author of *Draw Up a Chair: Short Stories to Inspire and Experience* and *The Colours of Virtue*

The BBC programme *Who Do You Think You Are?* reflects a society currently interested in family genealogy as a way of gaining guidance from our past and elucidation of our present. We gasp to see common physical attributes in photographs, shared interests in employment choices, and generations of birth patterns such as the production of non-identical twins, etc. But rather than viewing ourselves as victims of our past, Debbie's book helps us discover ourselves as energetic beings that have the power to take control of our present happiness and health.

Some readers may not have heard of the subtle energies — varying wavelengths beyond the physical dimension of time and space that help us experience different phenomena at several levels. However, all will be intrigued to discover that this energy field is a far greater source of information about our health than any other neurological or pathological source, as diseases may be seen there long before they manifest themselves physically. Read on if you want to learn how our emotional body bridges our physical and mental lives and how, because thoughts have power, we need to use them wisely. And enjoy meeting your spiritual body which transcends the physical and acts as a connector to our soul — that part of us that knows what is in our best interests and what is needed for our growth and development. But we not only exist in a world of energies, we do so in a liquid crystalline-structured state.

However, whilst the balance of the energy flow is controlled by a complex system of energy centres and pathways — the chakras and meridians — it may be influenced by the seven rays of light, karmic patterns and miasms that can contribute to ill health. But help is at hand. As an experienced complementary therapist, Debbie is able to demonstrate how 'energy medicines' such as flower and vibrational essences, can assist us in managing our multi-dimensional energetic self, embrace our innate intuitive faculties and higher wisdom and raise our light vibration. Thus, we not only learn who we really are, we discover how to become true and authentic by making decisions that will bring joy, contentment and good health now, despite what lies in the past.

Jan Stewart, Chair of the Confederation of Registered Essence Practitioners (COREP) and author of many books including *The Making of The Primary School* and *Exploring Primary Science and Technology with Microcomputers*

You Are a Frequency

How Personal Vibration Influences
Health, Well-Being and Development

You Are a Frequency

How Personal Vibration Influences
Health, Well-Being and Development

Debbie Anne Sellwood

BOOKS

Winchester, UK
Washington, USA

JOHN HUNT PUBLISHING

First published by O-Books, 2024
O-Books is an imprint of John Hunt Publishing Ltd., 3 East St., Alresford,
Hampshire SO24 9EE, UK
office@jhpbooks.com
www.johnhuntpublishing.com
www.o-books.com

For distributor details and how to order please visit the 'Ordering' section on our website.

ISBN: 978 1 80341 396 9
978 1 80341 397 6 (ebook)
Library of Congress Control Number: 2022922713

A CIP catalogue record for this book is available from the British Library.

Design: Lapiz Digital Services

UK: Printed and bound by CPI Group (UK) Ltd, Croydon, CR0 4YY
Printed in North America by CPI GPS partners

The author of this book does not dispense medical advice or
prescribe the use of any technique as a form of treatment for
physical, emotional, or medical problems without the advice of a
physician, either directly or indirectly. The intent of the author
is only to offer information of a general nature to help you in
your quest for emotional and spiritual well-being. In the event
you use any of the information in this book for yourself, which is
your constitutional right, the author and the publisher assume no
responsibility for your actions.

We operate a distinctive and ethical publishing philosophy in
all areas of our business, from our global network of authors to
production and worldwide distribution.

Contents

Preface 1

Acknowledgments 3

Introduction 5

Chapter 1 Energy, What and Who You Are 13

Chapter 2 The Subtle Anatomy — The Esoteric
Constitution of a Human 20

The Etheric Body 20

The Emotional Body 26

The Mental Body 37

The Soul 45

Chapter 3 The Body's Energy Network 56

Chapter 4 We Are All One 66

Chapter 5 We Are Crystals 72

Chapter 6 The Seven Rays of Light 83

Chapter 7 Is There a Reason or Purpose for Illness? 95

Chapter 8 Karma and Its Relationship to Health 101

Chapter 9 Miasms 106

Chapter 10 Solutions for Well-Being and the Way
Forward 114

Chapter 11 Are Energy Treatments the Future? 129

Chapter 12 It's All About Light 147

About the Author 159

Bibliography 160

Also by Debbie Sellwood
Centaury for Virgo, Rock Rose for Pisces, 2007
ISBN 978-1-905398-13-3

To Jack, Vinny, Ellamae, William, Dexter, Austin and Brodie.
May you hold the highest frequency and shine brightly on
your paths through life.

Preface

As a spiritual seeker for many years, one of my prime objectives, has been to understand who I am and what my path in life is from a spiritual perspective. The latter has been important in my role as an Astrologer and Flower Essence Practitioner especially in relation to helping others and their well-being, and it is this that has motivated me to write this book.

One of the most fundamental expectations of human existence is to be healthy in order to live a fulfilling life, yet the extent to which we consciously and unconsciously participate into our health status is not always appreciated. It is helpful to be conscious that everything is energy, and we as humans are no exception to this. We may appear to be physical, emotional and mental beings, but we also comprise of subtle energy, which expresses as our own unique frequency. This vibration can be 'tuned' to affect well-being in a positive way, or not according to the development of our consciousness. As humans we are the physical embodiment of our consciousness, including all the complexities involved in who we are emotionally, mentally and spiritually. Whilst many people are awakening to the importance of positively 'inputting' into their own health by managing their emotions and thoughts, and thus adjusting their vibration, this is still not an accepted theory for many including in medical circles.

With current health systems under pressure, and not often fully addressing individual needs, associated with a reliance in society on pharmaceutical drugs, a paradigm shift is waiting to happen. My book is relevant to these times as it describes the necessity and advantages of taking responsibility for one's health and in the most natural way possible.

In this book, I highlight the importance of this turbulent time in our history, and how our increasing awareness enables us to recognise our potential beyond purely identification with the physical body. A great amount of spiritual wisdom is resurfacing and much ancient knowledge, is now being revealed. We are at an opportune time to remember who we really are, what we are capable of being/doing and how we need to evolve in order to adjust to the future.

.

Acknowledgments

Finally, my second book has arrived after many years and much inner prompting, I could not ignore the whispers anymore. Thank you to my unseen help and guidance, without it there would be no book. My gratitude goes to Elizabeth Medler and Jan Stewart for their suggestions and support in writing this book. Thanks also to the authors who have imparted their wisdom in the many books I have read over the years, enabling me to consolidate my understanding in order to be able to write this book.

Introduction

A twenty-first-century spiritual perspective of the human constitution, body, and health potential from the perspective of subtle energy.

The twenty-first century is proving to be a momentous time in the Earth's history, providing many challenges, yet many blessings. Whilst humanity has always been influenced by cosmic energies, we are now experiencing a greater influx of energies which is accelerating our evolutionary process and initiating a new cycle of human existence. Humanity is being driven to understand and experience itself in a more expanded way; we are discovering we are far more than we thought. Whilst we navigate our path through these transformational times, it is crucial not only to acclimatise to these new energies but to also understand we are vibrating particles of energy ourselves and how to best manage this aspect of ourselves, especially in relation to our well-being. This is easier to achieve if we firstly understand who we really are at a more complete level.

One of the main objectives of this book is to explain that we are considerably more than just a physical body. The field of quantum physics has proved that everything in the universe is energy vibrating at different frequencies, even though it may look stationary. This is also true of humans. In addition to a physical body, we are also composed of subtle energies which operate at varying wavelengths beyond the physical dimension of time and space. Those unfamiliar with this description of human anatomy, may find it provocative as it requires perceiving oneself in a totally different way than envisioned before. Energy operates throughout every aspect of our ourselves (and our lives), including our health, the lack of which can also be ascribed to an energetic process. The condition of a human body is obviously dependent to a great extent on what is put into it, this means not just food and water, but the thoughts in our minds and the emotions we carry, which are also energy. The state of our consciousness has a significant bearing on our health and well-being, physically, emotionally, mentally and spiritually and explaining the importance of this is a major part of this book.

The physical body is the arena in which all human emotions play out, it shows us what needs healing. But do we have a system of health that supports this approach? Our current medical/health system is limited in various ways, many questions are now being raised around traditional medical practices, and the dominance and reliance on drugs. As it becomes more common place to view ourselves as energy beings, it will become increasingly apparent that our current health and medical systems are not adequate for their intended tasks. The author's belief is that we are entering a time when established healing methods and treatments will not only be less effective, but redundant. For many years we have been on the fringes of a new model of health care, one that acknowledges the necessity to approach healing from an appreciation of the 'whole person', not just the physical form. This means the inclusion of a subtle energy counterpart, as mentioned earlier. So far, however, it is mostly alternative and complementary therapies that have led the way and embraced this principle in their treatments, but this is changing. Although we can look forward to technological advances in health treatments, (some may likely arrive before the publication of this book[1]), taking responsibility for our own health and understanding more about what constitutes our well-being, will be key. In this book, I write about one aspect of energy treatment which is already established and flourishing.

To fully appreciate our 'whole being', we need to understand that the physical body alone does not provide the complete picture of who we are or what constitutes our health and well-being. The human form is surrounded by an electromagnetic energy field which is composed of a matrix of multi-dimensional energy bodies, known as the subtle energy system. It underlies, penetrates and surrounds the physical body and contributes to its operation and well-being. This energy field emits an individual frequency signature which provides a gauge as to how we are operating physically. The view that humans are more than just a physical body and emit an electromagnetic field, is an accepted theory in eastern medicine and in the western world of complementary medicine but is yet to be considered by traditional medical fields in the west. Our existence is multi-layered, and we need a system of medical care that reflects this.

One way to understand the basis of how our subtle anatomy works is to look at the model of the hologram, which can be described in very simple terms as a 3D photo made with a laser. If the photo were cut into pieces, the whole is mirrored within each of the many pieces; every piece contains the information of the whole. Richard Gerber M.D. (1954–2007) provides an understanding on how the hologram relates to our multi-dimensional configuration. He writes, 'The Hologram provides us with a new and unique model which may help science to understand the energetic structure of the universe as well as the multidimensional nature of human beings.'[2] A human comprises of a series of multi-dimensional subtle-energy systems that are all interacting with each other. Hence if every piece contains the whole, not only do components of our subtle energy systems contain complete knowledge of our physical bodies, every cell in our body is also a hologram, containing the pattern of the whole body and contributing to its condition.

To grasp how energy operates in relation to the human form, it is essential to understand how emotions and thoughts (including unconscious conditioning) are energies which can affect our health in either a supportive or adverse manner.

We are what we are because of energy, and the human body is a holographic projection of this consciousness. Many people are aware (especially with numerous books on this subject) of how mind and emotions contribute to our well-being, but the concept that our consciousness creates our reality has yet to fully infiltrate into mainstream medicine. The introduction of quantum physics in the early 1900s proved that the behaviour of energy at the quantum level is determined by the awareness of the observer, according to Einstein's principle 'energy comprises both a wave and particle form'. This means the future exists as an infinite array of possibilities and probabilities, the wave is a possibility of what could be, but it is not until we focus our attention on something or translate our idea into a thought, that it becomes manifest. The wave then changes from a state of potential to a state of being, it then becomes the particle, which, in the context of this book, is us and our corresponding state of health. Stem Biologist Bruce Lipton writes, 'At the atomic level, matter does not even exist with certainty; it only exists as a tendency to exist.'[3] Therefore, despite us perceiving our bodies as solid, matter and energy are interchangeable, in reality our bodies consist of nothing but slower energy presenting as solid form. In the quantum world, as we are both the observer and the creator of everything, this means we have far more involvement in the health of our bodies (and what happens to us generally) than we think. The future is not fixed, various options exist, every given moment contains unlimited promise for our future lives/health. We are able to influence the wave (the energy that has the potential for good or ill health) as to whether the body (a collection of particles) is healthy or not. It is our choice. We are moving away from the outdated paradigm that purports 'illness is done to one', we are beginning to realise, we are in control of who we are. Of course, there are exceptions, this statement does not address genetic illness, for example, mentioned later in the book.

Despite discovery of this quantum principle a hundred years ago, it is still not reflected in either mainstream consciousness or applied in medical practice. One of the reasons is because doctors are trained to view the body in accordance with Newtonian physics, as a physical machine where the different parts are not intimately interconnected. This contrasts with what scientists know about the invisible subatomic world and how everything is connected. Another reason is that it is not in the interests of certain organisations or companies that society is empowered in this way, hence we have been kept uninformed. Fortunately, many are now seeing through this illusion.

Progress moves slowly in the medical world and embracing health and well-being from the perspective of more ethereal forces, has not so far been considered, yet alone implemented. Not only do we need a system of health care that views humans as energetic beings, but one which cultivates a culture of self-responsibility, and where patients are empowered. The existing healthcare model where the doctor is the authority can often leave a patient feeling helpless and unable to contribute to the treatment/healing process. The reality is the patient is far from powerless, just lacking an understanding of how their consciousness can have a bearing on their subtle energy system which then ultimately influences their health. A future health paradigm will take into consideration the patient's contribution in situations of ill health, so that with some guidance and understanding, they can learn to recognise and offer an opinion as to which factors they feel may be contributing to the cause of their illness. It is hoped that this book will go some way in explaining how this works. Caroline Myss, internationally renowned speaker and author in the fields of human consciousness, spirituality, health, energy medicine and the science of medical intuition, sheds light on the importance of grasping our authority and taking responsibility for ourselves. She writes, 'The universal human journey is one of becoming conscious of our power and how to use that power. Becoming conscious of the responsibility inherent in the power of choice represents the core of this journey.'[4] 'Evaluating our beliefs is a spiritual and biological necessity. Our physical bodies, minds, and spirits all require new ideas in order to thrive.'[5]

As part of the human journey, we, and all life systems, experience constant change, we participate in a continual journey of evolution, this is an inevitable part of life. Growth is something we cannot avoid, it happens to us every day whether it is at a physical, emotional, mental or spiritual level. As we progress and develop into a greater functioning reality (ideally), we are often required to eliminate certain elements that no longer serve our highest good and incorporate other elements which will assist and further our evolution. Our purpose is to evolve, and as we do so our increased level of consciousness can contribute beneficially to our health. The nature of human evolution, as it pertains to changes to the physical form, is usually considered to occur over vast periods of time. According to science, the forces that create this change are natural selection and adaptation to the environment. However, influential and respected teacher of Esoteric Philosophy William Meader views this subject differently, 'However, the Esoteric Philosophy views this in a slightly different manner. Instead of seeing it as a physical event, it is understood as a dynamic process occurring within consciousness. It is consciousness that is evolving, and physical form will, over time, reflect these changes. The evolution of the physical body simply represents the adjustments that form naturally makes in response to the gradual changes occurring within the human psyche, which is quite different than the view held by the scientific community. Indeed, what science considers evolution, Esotericism sees as merely its effect.'[6] This statement sheds light on a person's ability to influence their physical body by changing their consciousness. Referring here to the subtle energetic system as vehicles, William continues, 'Spiritual evolution involves altering the chemistry of one's vehicles so that its substance becomes less dense and of a higher grade. This is done through the purification of the lower nature. Such change ultimately results in a healthier body, loftier emotions and a tendency towards elevated thought.'[7] The lower nature referred to by William refers to unhelpful emotions and behaviours that form the shadow side of our personalities. This book explores how by changing our consciousness we can move beyond our lower nature to constructively impact our well-being. I expand on this by explaining the process of how consciousness has a bearing on our energy bodies which ultimately influences our health.

From the author's perspective, one of the main purposes of life is to become conscious that we are more than a physical body with a personality but also a spiritual being experiencing physical life in material form. In this regard, I share my understanding of ancient esoteric knowledge and mention concepts such as the existence of the soul, past lives and karma. Additionally, I include the channelled writings (Djwhal Khul) of Alice Bailey (1880–1949), a theosophist and prolific author and of Gurudas, otherwise known as Ronald Lee Garman (1945–2001). Gurudas was an alternative health practitioner specializing in vibrational healing and radionics, an author and pioneer of herbs, flower, and gem essences and founder of an essence company. The material in his book,[8] from which I quote, was channelled with Kevin Ryerson, a professional psychic and trance medium.

In the first chapter, I present further explanation of our subtle energy system which can be defined as the receptacle for our consciousness, our holographic representation on the earth plane.

Endnotes

1. Prepare for Change (2022) Med Beds. Available at https://prepareforchange.net/?s=med+beds (Accessed: September 2022)

2. Gerber, R. (1996) *Vibrational Medicine. New Mexico:* Bear & Company Publishing, p. 45 3. Bruce Lipton quote. Available at http://www.grandhabit.com/quotes/bruce-lipton/v (Accessed: September 2022)

4. Myss, C. (1997) *Anatomy of the Spirit.* New York: Bantam, p. 110

5. Myss, C. (1997) *Anatomy of the Spirit.* New York: Bantam, p. 111

6. Meader, W. A. (2013) *The Evolution of Consciousness — Two Merge as One.* Available at: http://www.meader.org/2013/03/the-evolution-of-consciousness-two-merge-as-one/ (Accessed: September 2022)

7. Meader, W. A. (2004) *Shine Forth: The Soul's Magical Destiny,* California: Source Publications, p. 143

8. Gurudas. (1989) *Flower Essences and Vibrational Healing,* California: Cassandra Press

Chapter 1

Energy, What and Who You Are

If you want to find the secrets of the universe, think in terms of energy, frequency and vibration. **Nikola Tesla**[1]

Naturally, we are most familiar with the material world. This is because our senses are tuned to the physical realm, but in our 'extended self', we are actually existing in a higher spectrum of consciousness, on more than one plane of existence. In other words, we are spanning many realities, although most of us are unaware of this.

The physical plane vibrates at a lower level than other planes, hence its density in matter. Higher planes (where our other bodies exist) are composed of higher frequencies of energy. Planes can be seen to be organised according to varying frequencies, often referred to as dimensions or densities. These can be envisaged as states of consciousness or points of perception, rather than actual places. It could be that dimensions are sub-planes of planes, but discussing planes and dimensions is obviously entering into an area which is impossible to define. The author's description of these is based on her understanding, others may interpret these fields differently, or indeed the existence of such. Dimensions are the means by which we move our consciousness from one focus to another; we can be present simultaneously in other dimensions, but at varying degrees.

We live in the third dimension, thought by most people as the only reality existing, which is a very restricted and limited experience as it is based on beliefs such as judgement, duality and fear. Our concentration at the third dimensional level enables us to be able to use our five senses to experience the earth plane and communicate with others. Each dimension vibrates at a higher rate than the one below it[2] and it is thought that in each higher dimension we have access to a greater level of awareness and a wider perspective of reality. This enables us to experience more freedom, greater power and more opportunity to shape our reality. It should be noted that 'higher' dimensions are no better or worse than others, all have equal value and are considered essential to our varied life experiences.

As we only see a narrow band width of our actual reality, the average person is unaware that the physical body is not functioning in isolation but is enveloped in a spectrum of subtle bodies which exist and operate at higher vibrational levels. We (our total 'being') comprise of subtle bodies vibrating at varying wavelengths, but unlike the physical body, they are not visible to our eyes because of their higher rate of vibration. We know from physics, different frequencies can exist within the same space, and this is true for the physical body and its subtle body attachments, the only difference being their rate of vibration. Each subtle body exists in its own consciousness, functioning as a complete whole yet interconnected and interacting with the other bodies. This multi-dimensional energy field surrounds and permeates the physical form, extending a short distance around it. Collectively these bodies are commonly referred to as 'subtle bodies', 'subtle anatomy' or 'human energy field'. The subtle anatomy is an ethereal part of man's multi-dimensional self and the intermediary between the physical body and the life force energy (read about this in Chapter 2). These energy 'vehicles' consist of frequencies which enable one to interact on different levels of consciousness and their frequency of vibration determines the actual properties like shape and size of the matter they surround; this rate of vibration supplies us with our own unique energy signature. These complex energy fields interface with the cellular systems of the body and their condition can have a profound influence on the physical form, which vibrates at a far slower rate. It is probably more correct to visualise ourselves as an energy field which has the power to generate and orchestrate physical matter, rather than thinking of ourselves as a body with an energy field.

The existence of a subtle energy system surrounding a person is not as speculative as it sounds. Harold Saxon Burr (1889–1973) was E. K. Hunt Professor Emeritus of Anatomy at Yale University School of Medicine and an author.[3] He is most well known for his claim that all living things are moulded and controlled by invisible, intangible electro-dynamic fields of energy which he refers to as the Fields of Life, or L-fields, for short. Whilst at Yale, he accumulated a considerable amount of facts to support the hypothesis that these subtle energy fields govern the human body. He also discovered how they could be measured and mapped using standard voltmeters and electrodes and that changes in the electrical potential of the L-field would lead to changes in the health of the organism.[4]

Another scientist, Dr Fritz-Albert Popp (1938–2018), was a researcher in biophysics, particularly in Biophotonics, a branch of quantum biology. He conducted research that proves humans (and all biological organisms) emit frequencies of light and that even our metabolism depends on the function of light. He coined the term *biophoton* to describe these particles of light which transmit information within and between cells. His work shows that DNA in a living cell stores and releases photons creating 'biophotonic emissions' and that they may hold the key to illness and health. Dr Popp believed that this faint radiation, rather than biochemistry, is the true driving force in orchestrating and coordinating all cellular processes in the body. He theorized that this light must be like a master tuning fork setting off certain frequencies that would be followed by other molecules in the body. After years of comprehensive experimentation, Dr Popp demonstrated that these tiny frequencies were mainly stored and emitted from the DNA of cells and these signals contained valuable information about the state of the body's health.[5] His work suggests that healing may be a matter of reprogramming these quantum fluctuations, so they operate more coherently. In her book *Tuning the Diamonds: Electromagnetism & Spiritual Evolution*, Susan Joy Rennison refers to these quantum fluctuations, 'This light makes up the human energy field, commonly referred to as the aura.'[6]

The term *aura* is often used to describe the complete energy field which expands uniquely around each person and acts as a shield. The author's understanding is that it is a general term for the field of energies generated and emitted by the body, it reflects the metabolic and physiological processes of the body, whereas the subtle bodies are more specific electromagnetic energy fields. The electromagnetic rays of the auric field reveal the status of the physical and other subtle bodies.

The late Dr Valerie Hunt (1916–2014) was a scientist, neurophysiologist, author,[7] lecturer and Professor Emeritus of Physiological Science at the University of California, Los Angeles. She was best known for her pioneering research in the energy field, the form of light that radiates from the human body. She considered that the human energy field is the primary source of the interaction of a person with her/his environment in that whatever happens to one, it is this that is influenced ahead of anything in the nervous system or brain. She believed our energy field is a far greater source of information about the health of the body than any other neurological or pathological information derived from our chemistry of tissues. Her research uncovered that the energy field data carries one thousand to ten thousand greater frequency information per second than neurological frequency data. In an interview, advocating a rich, stable energy field is a healthy field, she stated, 'The energy fields of healthy people are coherent, synchronous, but unwell people's auras are demonstrably incoherent. What I have found by measuring people's auras is that disease begins in the energy field and anchors in the cells. If disease begins in the field, then health should also begin in the field. The field should be our place of primary diagnosis.'[8] 'Health first and foremost is health of the electromagnetic field. You're not going to have health if you don't have health in the electromagnetic field because this is the source.'[9]

Every cell and molecule in the human body has consciousness and when operating at optimal frequency is when they are vibrating at their highest rate, presumably as they were designed to. When this happens, there is harmony in the whole body resulting in perfect health. If an organ is healthy, its molecules are working together in a harmonious relationship with other organs but if disharmonious energies disturb this pattern, illness may become established. Diana Mossop, researcher into the healing properties of flower and plant essences and creator of her range of flower essences, Phytobiophysics®, sees the process in the following way, 'Every cell in the body vibrates on a frequency which is ordered and in harmony with the whole.... All elements, chemical substances, viruses and diseases vibrate on frequencies.... When substances block in the system they create a toxic load which vibrates on a disturbing frequency. Electromagnetic interference occurs in the nervous system which paralyses the nerve plexuses and causes lymphatic congestion and a breakdown of energy flow. Toxins which block in the lymphatic system also cause congestion and interfere with the energy flow. This interference automatically causes imbalance, disharmony and disease.'[10]

Everything is energy and energy is continuous, it never dies, it just transforms into another state; we are ongoing entities (as consciousness), whether we possess a physical body or not. Richard Gerber M.D. (1954–2007) considered this consciousness essential to the body. 'For truly, it is the endowing power of spirit that moves, inspires, and breathes life into that vehicle we perceive as the physical body. A system of medicine which denies or ignores its existence will be incomplete, because it leaves out the most fundamental quality of human existence — the spiritual dimension.'[11] The human energy field is a unified entity, the container for our consciousness and the equipment through which we experience other dimensions of reality. The elements which make up the energy field will be covered in the next chapter.

Energy is not created or destroyed, it can only be changed from one form to another. **Einstein**[12]

Endnotes

1. Nikola Tesla quote. Available at https://quotefancy.com/quote/11150/Nikola-Tesla-If-you-want-to-find-the-secrets-of-the-universe-think-in-terms-of-energy#:~:text=Nikola%20Tesla%20Quote%3A%20%E2%80%9CIf%20you (Accessed: September 2022)

2. I use 'below' and 'higher' to make it easy to understand although I imagine it is not necessarily that straightforward.

3. Burr, H. S. (1972) *The Fields of Life: Our links with the Universe.* New York: Ballantine Books

4. Walker, P. F. *Harold Saxton Burr.* Available at http://www.blissviews.wordpress.com/harold-saxton-burr/

5. International Union of Medical and Applied Bioelectrography (2018) *Prof. Fritz Albert Popp.* Available at http://www.iumab.org/prof-fritz-albert-popp/ (Accessed: September 2022)

6. Rennison, S. J. (2008) *Tuning the Diamonds: Electromagnetism & Spiritual Evolution.* 2nd edition. England: Joyfire Publishing. p. 93

7. Hunt, V. (1996) *Infinite Mind: Science of the Human Vibrations of Consciousness.* USA: Malibu Publishers

8. Freshmag (2016) *The Science of human vibrations.* Available at http://www.freshmag.com.au/human-vibrations-science/ (Accessed: September 2022)

9. Triv, L. (2012) *The Human Energy Field: An Interview with Valerie V. Hunt, Ph.D.* Available at http://www.healthontheedge.wordpress.com/2012/01/28/the-human-energy-field-an-interview-with-valerie-v-hunt-ph-d/ (Accessed: September 2022)

10. Mossop, D. (1997) *The Power of Plants.* Jersey, UK: The Institute of Phytobiophysics p. 3

11. Gerber, R. (1996) *Vibrational Medicine. New Mexico:* Bear & Company Publishing p. 419

12. Einstein quote. Available at https://www.goodreads.com/quotes/4455-energy-cannot-be-created-or-destroyed-it-can-only-be (Accessed: November 2022)

Chapter 2

The Subtle Anatomy — The Esoteric Constitution of a Human

The Etheric Body

We are still on the threshold of fully understanding the complex relationship between light and life, but we can now say emphatically, that the function of our entire metabolism is dependent on light.
Dr Fritz Albert Popp[1]

The etheric body is one component of the subtle anatomy. It is situated closest to the physical body, extends a short distance from it and has several responsibilities. One of its tasks is to act as a framework for the physical body, so our outer form is modelled on it. It acts like a scaffold, holding the physical body together as an integral whole otherwise without it we would just be a collection of independent cells. It is often referred to as an 'energy double' being a replica or mirror image of every cell, tissue, organ or part of the physical body. It is thought to contain a model of the whole human body but contains the pattern to organise and maintain its molecular and cellular systems. In *Vibrational Medicine*, Richard Gerber M.D. (1954–2007) writes, 'The etheric body is a holographic energy template that guides the growth and development of the physical body. Distortions of the healthy pattern of subtle-energy organization in the etheric template may lead to abnormal cellular growth. From what is known about the etheric body, diseases appear to be seen in the etheric field weeks and months prior to their becoming manifest in the physical body.'[2]

It is intriguing to know we have a doppelgänger, yet most people are unaware of this unseen but necessary attachment to the physical body. In fact, it is vital to our existence as it is the etheric that generates the physical body. The physical form is completely dependent on the existence of the etheric body, which has been in existence since our birth, if the etheric no longer exists, neither does the physical body. Humans are not unique in possessing an etheric body, all living things including the Earth have one. William Meader explains, 'Everything densely physical has etheric substance underlying it and providing energetic support for its manifested existence. Outer forms cannot exist without this foundation of etheric substance.'[3] Rupert Sheldrake, Ph.D., biologist, author and researcher in the field of parapsychology, is most renowned for his theory on morphic resonance. He proposes there is a developmental energy field within and around a morphic unit (which he defines as a cell, tissue, organ or organism, etc.) and the field actually forms it. Through morphic resonance these units develop according to the programmes within that field. He writes, 'Morphic fields, like the known fields of physics such as gravitational fields, are nonmaterial regions of influence extending in space and continuing in time. They are localized within and round the systems they organize.'[4]

We are aware that in order to survive in life there are a few basic measures which must be adhered to on a regular basis. For instance, we cannot exist without breathing oxygen, eating, drinking, exercising to some degree and being exposed to light. Yet these activities alone are not sufficient to sustain the physical body which also relies on a life force energy to nourish, support and maintain it. We know the Sun radiates light and heat, but its other emission is that of etheric energy, known by different cultures as Qi (or Ch'i), Ka, Mana or Prana. I will use the word Prana in the text from now on. These waves of universal life energy are all around us, permeating all of space; they stream through all living things, giving life to them. It appears some sort of mystical process takes place where the body is filled with this light which is subsequently transformed into life force energy. Often known as etheric energy, Prana is not to be confused with oxygen, which is a gas, but it is thought that this subtle energy is carried in oxygen molecules.

The concept that everything in nature is permeated by energy, was intrinsic to the philosophies of ancient civilisations such as China, Japan and India, and remains so today. They have always instinctively understood that everything in nature is infused with life-giving energy and without it nothing would exist. This concept of vibrant life energy is a vital principle, fundamental in several systems of complementary medicine, such as acupuncture, kinesiology, crystal healing, and vibrational essence therapy, where energy in the body is balanced or enhanced. The principle of moving energy is also employed in the practice of Yoga, Tai Ch'i, and Qigong and is passed to recipients in healing modalities such as Reiki or Spiritual Healing.

The etheric body receives and serves as a channel for this vital energy flowing from the Sun, Prana is absorbed by all living organisms. It provides fuel (the body's heat and maintenance), a sufficient supply of which is essential in vitalising the etheric and subsequently the physical body. The etheric body, acts as a receiver and assimilator, storing up rays of light from the Sun and maintaining a reservoir of life energy. This energy, received by the etheric body (after being modified into a form that is acceptable for it to receive) exerts a specific vibratory rate onto the physical form, keeping it preserved, repaired and in a vitalised condition. When sunlight is plentiful, Prana is more abundant, but at night its deficiency means we feel the need for sleep and while we do so we recharge from the supply within the etheric body and the etheric charged atmosphere around us. When the sky is cloudy, etheric energy is reduced, explaining why some people become low or depressed on grey days.

It is the role of the etheric body to ensure the physical body resides in an orderly and healthy state and because both bodies are energetically connected, any imbalance in the etheric body, ultimately affects the physical form. Since the performance of the physical body is totally dependent on the condition of the etheric body, an uninhibited flow of Prana is essential to keeping all aspects of the physical body working well and preserving good health. Alice Bailey emphasises this, 'It is of course apparent that where there is a free flow of force through the etheric body into the dense physical body there will be less likelihood of disease or sickness.'[5] How the physical body registers and reacts to these energies is important, the quality of the impressions received can vary in vibration and quality according to the status of the receiving etheric body. Hence, if its condition is strong, these energies are not restricted, the etheric is able to function with resilience. If it absorbs sufficient high-quality Prana which keeps the physical body orderly and the organs working correctly, the etheric is able to do its job correctly and protect us from illness. If, however, the reverse is true (the etheric body is deficient) it therefore cannot transmit Prana effectively or sufficiently; it is not functioning optimally. In this case, the frequency of the energy received is lowered and devitalised which, over a period of time, can reduce the efficiency of the immune system, ultimately impairing physical health.

The purer and more refined the status of the receiving etheric body, the more proficient the receiver of Prana it is, hence the healthier the body will be. So how can we ensure we receive unimpeded Prana, and have a healthy etheric body? A healthy lifestyle and a good diet are key as our bodies absorb Prana from elements that contain it such as food and water. So, eating unadulterated, organic foods and drinking pure spring water is important. As the atoms in our bodies are constantly replaced by food, water and air, the etheric body is also changed (or charged) by these elements and by Prana. Air is filled with etheric energy, and this is especially so when the sun is shining, so being outside and breathing good quality air is essential. Living in an area where the air is clean, fresh, and unpolluted, is to our benefit. We can also enable the best possible condition of the etheric body if our intentions and motives are of the highest integrity, and we avoid worrying, stress and hanging on to detrimental emotions, the vibrations of which can disturb the equilibrium of this body and the other subtle bodies (discussed in detail in following chapters). In addition, awareness and control of one's breath is said not only to create more energy and enhance the immune system but create beneficial brain wave patterns. Barbara Marciniak, an internationally acclaimed trance channel, inspirational speaker and bestselling author writes, 'You can focus the energy of your breath with any imagery you like, according to how you want to feel or express yourself. Vital energy is free and completely open to be directed and moulded by you. When you consciously breathe, you immediately alter the frequency of your brain wave patterns into a more awakened and integrated state of awareness.'[6] This probably explains why Yogis place so much emphasis on breathing, they know a thing or two!

The etheric body (which resides on the etheric plane) is itself composed of etheric energy, a network of fine interlacing channels which protects the physical body against harmful radiation. It is also the divider between the physical and subtle bodies. It is not only responsive to forces from the environment (such as Prana), but another part of its complex responsibilities is that it serves as a medium for the transmission of energies to the rest of the subtle anatomy. It interacts and reacts to the energies of the other subtle bodies and their condition; everything that happens to the etheric is conveyed energetically to other parts of this system and ultimately the physical body. This intricate interweaving and network of energies will be discussed in a following chapter.

When there is a free flow of energy from the etheric into the physical body there is less chance of illness occurring, although there are other factors such as the condition of the other subtle bodies. An example is the emotional body which is connected with our emotions, and I explain more in the next chapter. Biophysicist and energy medicine pioneer Beverley Rubik, PhD. refers to her previous paper, *The Biofield Hypothesis*, when she writes the following. 'I wrote it in 2002, and in it I stated that the biofield is electromagnetic, within and around the body. But today I would like to add that it is beyond that as well. I think of the biofield as an organizing field of life that reaches into the metaphysical domains of mind and spirit as well as the physical domain of electromagnetism, which is an invisible energy field governing how the cells and molecules of life respond, which regulates our physiology, that literally regulates our organism. But the conductor of this symphony of fields is the mind, and even above that the conductor is probably the emotions and at some level the soul and spirit. And, of course, as a scientist, here I am delving into metaphysics, and I am well aware of that.'[7]

The subtle physical body is made up of strands of luminous energy, and the energies are flowing through them constantly in the etheric plane. Above the subtle body is the causal body. **Fredrick Lenz**[8]

The Emotional Body

Every human being is the author of his own health or disease.
Buddha[1]

Many people are aware that our moods and the way we think can have a major impact on how we feel physically. At times, the intensity of our emotions can feel almost like an out-of-body experience, which is not surprising because our emotions and thoughts have their own (subtle) bodies. Whereas we are most familiar with the earth plane in which the physical body functions, the emotional body resides on the emotional plane, (read about planes and dimensions in Chapter 1) and has a natural affinity to the fourth dimension. This dimension holds an expression of our personality and is related to emotions, inner feelings, intuition and imagination. It is said to be the realm of the collective mind and can be experienced from a lower or higher outlook. If we are experiencing fear, for example, we are tuning into a lower fourth dimensional consciousness and our fear is likely to be magnified as we are vibrating with millions of others who are also experiencing this emotion. Whereas, if we are aligned to a higher fourth dimensional consciousness, we don't react unconsciously, we have more control over our emotions and feelings which are experienced as more flowing and with ease. Our focus is on what is happening in this minute, we operate in the 'Now'. The fundamentals of Eckhart Tolle's book *The Power of Now*[2] explain the dynamics of this concept.

In recent years, especially in relation to complementary healing, there has been greater emphasis on encouraging people to look within themselves in order to recognise and release intense destructive emotions, the withholding or suppression of which can cause havoc not only emotionally, but often physically. This focus has been attempting to move people out of a solely third dimensional outlook which does not entertain looking at things deeply. A deeper appreciation is more of a fourth dimensional view which awakens us to the idea that there is more to things on the surface of life than meets the eye. Along with this perspective comes an increase in intuition, a healthier approach to the way we live our lives, to the environment and the desire to find meaning and purpose in one's life.

The emotional body exists along with the other subtle bodies in a hierarchical system, with those furthest away from the physical body having the highest energetic frequencies. Whilst the etheric body vibrates at a higher frequency than the physical body, the emotional body has a higher frequency than the etheric body, the mental body a higher frequency than the emotional body, the soul body even higher and so on. These latter two bodies will be discussed in following sections in this chapter. There are yet higher energetic bodies than these, operating in other dimensions and inputting into the human experience, but these are not within the scope of this book.

The condition and functioning of the emotional body, (and mental body covered in the next section), are paramount to our well-being, and one of our life tasks is to acquire mastery over them both. The emotional body (sometimes known as the astral body) participates in our emotional expression and is the basis of our desires, wishes, impulses and behaviours; it is the source of every feeling we have, such as love, hate, fear or anger. When we partake in an activity that is agreeable, feelings of pleasure, happiness or enjoyment are evoked in this body, yet a less pleasurable activity may arouse an assortment of different feelings ranging from stress, frustration, discontent and boredom, each having different reactions in this body. When emotions of a more volatile nature, such as fear, hate and anger are constantly and strongly experienced, these are not supportive of a balanced emotional body and may over time be instrumental in generating a detrimental physical effect. The word 'e-motion' suggests a kind of activity or movement, our emotional states are exactly this, energy in motion. Dr David Hawkins M.D., Ph.D. (1927–2012) believed they equate to different frequencies of energy. He was a renowned psychiatrist, physician, researcher, spiritual teacher and lecturer and held that there is a hierarchy to the levels of human consciousness.[3] After testing thousands of people using kinesiology, he assigned a value in a logarithmic scale to levels of consciousness (from low to high). These are shame, guilt, apathy, grief, fear, desire, anger, pride, courage, neutrality, willingness, acceptance, reason, love, joy, peace and enlightenment. Whilst it can be normal to experience one or other of these states at certain points in our day, usually one state will dominate. An emotion such as shame has a value of 20, whilst peace is 600, but remember the relationship between these numbers is not linear but logarithmic.[4] This calibration of emotions probably confirms what most of us know, peace and joy are far healthier emotions to experience. It is in our best interest to ensure our emotional body is calm, so as to provide a sense of emotional stability and psychological security. In this way it will also be operating in harmony with the rest of the subtle anatomy, which is essential for our well-being.

We know that when we feel contented emotionally, this can also have an extraordinary effect on any physical incapacities; however, the medical establishment are slow to accept that emotions can affect health. Fortunately, science caught up many years ago with what many complementary therapies advocate, which is energy follows thought; your body is a manifestation of what you believe. Unfortunately, science does not seem to communicate fully with the medical establishment, but hopefully this is changing. In 1998, the work of Dr Candace Pert[5] brought a scientific approach to understanding how the mind and the body work together. In her capacity as a neuroscientist, and after decades of research, she was able to demonstrate that when we express an emotion it shows up in the body as a pattern of peptides (chemical messengers) which link to appropriate receptors (receivers of these messages) in various organs and muscles of the body and affect their function and produce a reaction. In other words, you are what you think and feel; you create your physical reality. This field of science is known as Psycho-Neuro-Immunology (PNI).

More recently Bruce Lipton, stem biologist and internationally recognised leader in bridging science and spirit, explains[6] that a new type of science called Epigenetics is growing in popularity and promise in the scientific world. Epigenetics means 'control above genetics' and it is the study of how behaviour, and external and environmental factors (such as upbringing and our experiences), turn our genes on and off, and in turn, define how our cells actually read those genes. Whereas in the original scientific paradigm it was believed that genes determine the character of our lives, this science demonstrates that it is the character of our lives that controls our genes. This means DNA does not predetermine how we are going to think, act or feel (well or ill), we are not predisposed to be of a certain disposition. It is our perception of what has happened to us that determines our reality and is instrumental in defining who we think we are, our aspirations in life and how we behave. We can influence our genes by changing our thoughts and emotions, which are subsequently translated by the body (PNI) into biochemical information. Of course, our assessment of what happens to us will be different from that of others according to the state of consciousness from which we are choosing to observe. The discovery of Epigenetics is important because whenever we have undergone an experience, we put our own perspective on it, whether it is true or not and whether it is detrimental to us, or not. This would imply we no longer need to be held hostage by our negative views and expectations. No wonder Bruce describes this science as self-empowering. Epigenetics and PNI are closely related, Epigenetics is the science behind how emotions can change our cells and PNI is the science behind how emotional and other psychological states (and hormones) have a physical repercussion on the body and the immune system.

Neale Donald Walsch, author and modern-day spiritual messenger reminds us, 'Quantum physics tells us that nothing that is observed is unaffected by the observer. That statement, from science, holds an enormous and powerful insight. It means that everyone sees a different truth, because everyone is creating what they see.'[7] This science aligns with the belief of quantum biologists that things don't become real until we look at or focus our attention on them. If we want good health, then we should be focusing on this with everything we have!

It is thought that illness and dis-ease can originate from a withholding or suppression of past hurts, squashing of emotions, unfulfilled desires, perceived inadequacies or disappointments such as the inability to realise one's goals. Illnesses may represent unexpressed feelings so it is imperative we do not quash or deny our feelings, these must be expressed in a healthy manner. Other reasons that may contribute to poor health may be the failure to remove undesirable influences from our lives or ignore issues that impact our happiness and well-being. So too must we honour our own sense of power and make sure it is expressed in a positive and constructive way. Our upbringing can leave within us a powerful legacy, but sadly it is not always the best. In this case, it can be typical in childhood, to develop patterns of behaviour in order to cope with experiences of trauma, abuse, mistreatment, negative reactions from others or just difficult life situations which can be carried throughout our life. In these circumstances, a survival instinct kicks in, and we often adopt a 'learned' response in order to protect ourselves. This may consist of feeling and expressing a variety of emotions ranging from anger, aggression, fear, jealousy, control, envy, denial or complete avoidance. This can also happen if we are 'programmed' by family or our social environment to behave in a way that is not true to who we fundamentally are at our core. We can unconsciously adopt family beliefs or behaviours, unwittingly repeating them and committing ourselves to a reality that has been informed by others. If we have been exposed to detrimental or damaging conditioning throughout childhood, this stores within us energetic patterns of frustration, anger and sometimes resignation, which if not resolved and released, can be toxic to health. We may feel powerless to do anything to change these conditions especially if we are enmeshed in a family where over concern for others means our boundaries are vulnerable. A situation like this or where we feel that we have to capitulate to beliefs that are consistent with those around us, discourages autonomous development and keeps one locked in an unhealthy situation. Even if our childhood was generally happy, we may still need to overcome beliefs handed down to us by family and society, which do not resonate with our true selves.

Continually reinforcing dysfunctional emotions, produces a dissonant frequency in the emotional body, often creating further congestion or disruption where energy is hindered and unable to flow smoothly. This blocked energy then affects the functioning of other components of the subtle anatomy including the etheric body, ultimately filtering to the physical body, and taking up residence as a physical problem. We may carry layers upon layers of destructive emotions which can hamper the body's immune system and natural healing ability. Memories, traumas and emotions can become trapped in parts of our bodies, which when left unresolved commits one to a situation where Prana and messages from the subtle anatomy are not properly received as the body is not functioning optimally. Alice Bailey writes, 'A man is, upon the physical plane, emotionally and mentally what his glandular system makes him, and incidentally what they make him physically, because that is frequently determined by his psychological state of mind and emotions.'[8]

Susan Joy Rennison describes emotions as *measurements*. 'Feelings and emotions are reactions to situations based upon the *interpretation* of the events. They are mirrors that allow you energetically to respond to and become aware of your own calibration to an event or experience.'[9] Measurements is a helpful word to use when evaluating the distressing repercussions of emotions which may have become profoundly embroiled in one's psyche. Does the extent to which we experience the effects of harmful emotions and feelings warrant hanging onto them? The answer is likely to be no. Whilst it can be difficult to change recently adopted behaviours, it is even more so to change deeply indoctrinated ones which may have been unknowingly informing one's beliefs and actions. It requires great courage to firstly, recognise unhealthy past conditioning or unresolved emotions that may not be in one's best interests. Secondly, to have the motivation to change or unlearn detrimental habits and thirdly, to rally the commitment to embark upon a path which involves healing/resolving these aspects. Whatever the experience, learning to release blocked feelings is not only in the best interests of one's health, but vital to a fulfilling future. In Chapter 11, 'Are Energy Treatments the Future?', I suggest natural ways of emotional healing.

In her book, Susan Joy Rennison refers to studies from the HeartMath Institute[10] when feelings of unconditional love, forgiveness and acceptance are constantly evoked, these are profound healers and re-establish balance and harmony in all our bodies. Yet, it is also not helpful to possess an overly compassionate and sensitive nature as this creates an emotional body that can become out of balance with the other subtle bodies. If our inclination is to constantly respond to life from an excessively emotional standpoint, this is likely to mean insufficient control over this body, resulting in it dominating the other bodies and creating imbalance between them. When there is turbulence in the emotional body, this creates a knock-on effect, setting up turmoil in the corresponding solar plexus chakra which is seen as a clearing house for emotions, (read more about the chakras in Chapter 3, 'The Body's Energy Network') and inharmoniously impacts the etheric body.

We may not be conscious of it, but we are constantly yet unknowingly affecting our emotional body, in an advantageous or harmful way. Striving for greater restraint over our emotions and subsequently changing destructive attitudes means more control over this body, thus preventing compromising the physical body. Biochemist Sondra Barrett Ph.D. advocates treating the cells in our bodies as sacred. She shares the results of a study evaluating stress hormones in the blood of a couple having had an argument. The woman continued to re-live the argument, hence her stress hormones remained elevated longer than her man's. Sondra writes, 'This study is a great reminder to let go of a stressful situation once we've experienced it in "real time." If we relive it over and over, we put our bodies, and their trillions of cell sanctuaries, in great distress. We risk illness and fatigue when our cells are thrown out of balance in this way. And we have a choice. While our cells are always in the now, our thoughts can sentence them to reliving *yesterday's* now.'[11] This last sentence is a powerful statement, serving to remind us that we have a choice. We only penalise ourselves by continually hanging onto and energising unhelpful emotions which are best released and forgotten. Our cells (which ideally are vibrating to a high frequency) are intelligent, so why sabotage our health by doing this? Sondra suggests we consider our cells as the sacred vessels of our lives and to bathe them in molecules of peacefulness and contentment, in the chemistry of love. Perfect, give your cells a break!

Most of us are 'work in progress' when it comes to managing our emotions. The emotional body is the most difficult to control, especially if mood swings and volatility is our norm; we can be driven by unconscious feelings. Maintaining self-control of our emotions is difficult when memories from our past are stored in our subtle anatomy, we can become unduly influenced, even obsessed with them. This can be true of both past and previous life events. Internationally acclaimed spiritual teacher and healer Chris Griscom referring to intense and traumatic experiences, writes, 'These traumas are biochemically and electromagnetically stored within the matrix of the emotional body. The imprint is carried along like an electrical impulse by the emotional body into each incarnation.'[12] This suggests when we come into a lifetime we can be hampered in our plans and aspirations by a collection of stored up emotional memories and unconscious reactions, which are demanding some sort of resolution before we can live our lives with fulfilment and to its maximum potential. Yet we are not usually consciously aware of this. A perpetual cycle can unfold where we encounter people or/ and circumstances (including maybe a health issue) of a similar nature, linked to the original experience. Chris writes that the emotional body is unable to differentiate between the past, present and future and magnetically attracts those experiences that are in its frame of reference. If we don't break free of these types of unsupportive habits, patterns and behaviours, we are likely to continue to experience similar situations or find, if we project them (usually unknowingly), they will be triggered (unhelpfully) by others expressing them for us. In which case we still have to deal with them. In her book, Janet McClure (d 1990),[13] a professional channel, uses the useful analogy of holding onto negative emotions as trying to spin plates on sticks. She believed that when unresolved emotional issues build up, this results in spinning a lot of plates. If an issue is resolved, the plate spins in balance eternally, but if not, we are continually giving attention to and wasting precious energy on plates left spinning and needing to be balanced. Unless you are in training for the circus, let go of those old, chipped, and wobbly plates! It is time to reclaim the energy which has been devoted to keeping highly charged emotions from the past, alive. We are so much more than our history; it is in our best interests not to let it dictate our future.

According to spiritual teachings and planetary/astrological cycles, functioning from the standpoint of our emotions is believed to have been the dominant and overriding phase for humans for a large part of our history. This stage of focusing our consciousness upon and developing our emotional bodies has been an important development for humanity in the past but has led unfortunately to selfishness, thoughts of a lower mind quality and materialistic desires, which has been a continuing trend until recently. Although in its infancy, a new cycle is beginning where humanity is awakening to their spiritual selves, we are now passing from a time where humans have been predominantly emotional and desire orientated, to a time where we are becoming more mentally aware, yet heart based. As humanity's consciousness is rising, it is also gaining greater understanding over how its thoughts create reality. This is not an overnight transformation and will not be effective until more people have greater cognisance of themselves as more than physical beings, and how it is desirable to be centred in the soul, (read more about the Soul in Chapter 2) rather than the personality. Planetary cycles govern long periods of time during which humans are subjected in various ways to constant change; all of which is instrumental in their continual evolution. A beneficial consequence of our current stage is that a great number of people are realising they need to take more responsibility for controlling their emotions, detaching and rising above and uplifting them when necessary. It is to our advantage to leave destructive emotions behind; they are not only a constraint to our current and future well-being but to that of subsequent generations (read about miasms which are a predisposition to various physical illnesses and conditions in Chapter 9). An unforeseen benefit to healing ourselves can result in healing those around us too. I write more about the relevance of these cycles upon our current stage of development in Chapter 6, 'The Seven Rays of Light'.

We may not be able to physically see what impact destructive emotions are having internally on our bodies, but our energy field reflects this. Susan Joy Rennison reminds us, 'When we work specifically with our emotional nature, we are also working with our electromagnetic nature, more specifically, the magnetic field emitted by the physical body.'[14] Dr Valerie Hunt writes, 'Then there is the question of coherency or stability, which has to do with whether the field comes back to a resting state when it's not being challenged. When the field starts to disintegrate or become anti-coherent, it means that things don't go together. You will have frequencies out of sync and the energy does not flow.... When we shift human emotion, we can do amazing things with the electromagnetic field.'[15] It is vital to process blocked emotions and move through upsets and rebalance as quickly as possible. It is our choice; we expand or limit our potential (on many levels) by the way we choose to handle our emotions.

When we learn to step back and observe how we are reacting, we become more conscious of our emotions, and our responses become more considered and neutral. In doing this, we are becoming experts at working with energy, specifically in favourably influencing our energy fields. Are you your best authority or do you allow others (now or from the past) to influence you? Do harmful emotions determine how you feel or behave? Do you choose calm in your life by having control over your emotions? You have the ability to decide whether you wish to be empowered or remain a casualty of your emotions. In the next chapter I describe the mental body.

What you think, you become. What you feel, you attract. What you imagine, you create. **Buddha**[14]

The Mental Body

All that we are is the result of what we have thought. **Buddha**[1]

The mental body is constructed of our thoughts. The structure of our ideas and mental processes takes place here and provides us with the capacity to visualise, consider concepts and ideas, to think rationally and make judgements. It is thought the mental body resides on the lower level of the mental plane and is most attuned to the fifth dimension. This dimension holds the creative potential, (the building blocks) for our physical existence which enables us to define our reality. When we become more conscious of working in this dimension, we begin to take responsibility for our reality by creating and choosing our experiences on earth.

Similar to our feelings and emotions, our thoughts, attitudes, beliefs and intentions are energy and according to their frequency have the ability to affect our well-being. Whenever we think about something or someone, we create energy, so it is impossible to think without some accompanying feeling, reaction or emotion. Our emotions are created by our thoughts; the mental body gives form to our feelings, so both the emotional and mental bodies are closely connected. A thought in itself is unlikely to be physically harmful. However, when it is impregnated with strong emotions, this makes it powerful and potentially damaging. The greater the emotional force fuelling a thought, the more effective it will be, for good or ill. It appears that even in biblical times, this was acknowledged, 'For as he thinketh in his heart, so *is* he' (Proverbs 23:7). Joan Hodgson, (1913–1995) who developed Astrology correspondence courses and was an author of several books, believed that in ancient times people understood that everything physical is connected to activities on higher planes and this is demonstrated by spiritual laws that govern our universe. She writes about one such law, 'The Law of Correspondences, whereby the state of our inner consciousness gradually and inevitably externalises itself in the physical body.'[2] In other words 'thought creates reality'. Perhaps there is a lot of wisdom in the old proverb 'A healthy mind lives in a healthy body'.

Although thoughts of a discouraging and pessimistic nature are not particularly helpful to our general spirits, they do not have the same amount of power as those that are continually fired by emotions such as hopelessness, fear or hate. If thoughts are imbued with toxic emotions, this can restrict the circulation of vibrant etheric energy; creating energetic obstructions in the entire subtle anatomy system, which can eventually affect the physical body in a detrimental way. Dr Pert's research (read the previous section on the Emotional Body) reveals that biochemicals carry messages of our thoughts and emotions throughout our bodies, leading to the conclusion that there is no separation between the mind and the body. Our consciousness creates and maintains the energetic blueprint (etheric body) which is responsible for the condition of bodily functions and overall maintenance of our bodies. It is imperative that what we believe about ourselves is complimentary because our bodies are a projection of this consciousness. If we can recognise disparaging, long suffering or critical thoughts towards ourselves, we are also able to change these beliefs, thus changing the energetic blueprint, the energy that underlies the human body.

Each time we have a thought, an energetic 'thought form' is created which vibrates to a certain frequency and has the potential to impact on events or what comes into reality, i.e., 'energy follows thought'. It is within the mental body that the creative process of thoughtform building takes place and is then communicated for possible action, to the brain. The mental body is the real thinker whilst the brain is the processor and transmitter of thoughts, in reality the tool of the mental body.

This observation that the mind extends beyond the brain was proposed by French mathematician and philosopher René Descartes (1596–1650) and is held by several scientists. Rupert Sheldrake suggests 'the mind stretches out through fields I call morphic fields'.[3] Morphic fields were defined in the section on the Etheric Body, in Chapter 2.

Lynne McTaggart, an international author, journalist, lecturer and integrative medicine activist explores the mind extending beyond the brain in greater detail in her book. She refers to Karl Pribram (1877–1973), a neurophysiologist. 'After Pribram's discoveries, a number of scientists, including systems theorist Ervin Laszlo, would go on to argue that the brain is simply the retrieval and read-out mechanism of the ultimate storage medium — The Field.'[4] She continues, 'If they are correct, our brain is not a storage medium but a receiving mechanism in every sense, and memory is simply a distant cousin of ordinary perception.'[5] This description seems to fit with the concept of the mental body located on a plane other than the physical. However, as a non-scientist, who does not wish to veer into more complicated descriptions, I will leave it there, but it does appear that there is a lot more going on with our minds than that which is located between our ears!

What we think about most often is what we are likely to bring into manifestation, so it is important to be conscious and use our ability to create thoughts wisely. If we continue to think a negative thought, we will likely bring into our reality, a negative outcome. We are solely responsible for what happens to us, and this is explained by the Law of Karma, 'what goes around, comes around'. Read more about Karma in Chapter 8. It is possible to change undesirable situations by changing our thoughts and perceptions of, for example, events, situations and people using positive reinforcement and expectation, visualisation and affirmation. We attract into our lives only circumstances and people that are attuned to our individual vibration. This is the basis of another spiritual law, the Law of Attraction, and there are many books written on this topic. It is not sufficient just to think positively about what one wants (in the context of this book, think good health) as positive thinking is a function of the conscious brain, whereas beliefs, thoughts and emotions of a negative nature are likely to be deeply ingrained in the unconscious and can be influencing us inadvertently. These unconscious emotions and feelings, which may need to be re-framed and reprogrammed, must be aligned on the same vibrational level as a positive thought-making process, in order for the thought to produce a successful outcome. We need to be realistic, however, as we don't always get what we think we need, but we often get what we require for our future growth. Read about Karma in Chapter 8. Whether we are trying to clear negative thoughts, dysfunctional behaviours or undertake self-healing, the intention (vibration) behind the emotion and thought, is crucial to success.

Barbara Brennan, a pioneer and innovator in the field of energy consciousness, has been working with the human energy field for more than thirty-five years. In *Light Emerging* she writes that the greatest implication over the state of our health is how we express our consciousness. She emphasises the primary factors as being how our intentions, both conscious and unconscious, are expressed in our thinking and feelings, and how these affect our auric field, as being the fundamental factors in health or dis-ease. She believes that the true dis-ease behind a physical manifestation is consciousness and the science and health care systems that focus on the physical are basing their assumptions on secondary, not primary causes.

The reality of what we experience in life is likely to equate to what we believe, yet it is not always easy to change a pattern of thinking which is not to our advantage. As a result of experiencing traumas or harsh childhood programming, some people can lose the ability to relate to their feelings. If we are polarised in the mental body, we are disconnected from our emotions which can result in being driven unconsciously, often to our detriment. The power of damaging unconscious programming cannot be underestimated for the subconscious mind is often dominant. Bruce Lipton writes, 'Subconscious programming takes over the moment your conscious mind is not paying attention.'[7] The words of Beatriz Singer, an expert on crystals, are of a similar theme, 'The unconscious mind can't distinguish between an imagined event and a real one. In our brains' energy fields — in which all experiences, real or imagined, are reduced to organized waveforms-our memories and imagination can play just as big a role as an actual event.'[8] However, we need to take back control in whichever way we can, as it is in our best interests to cleanse detrimental patterns and transform limited beliefs. If not, we chance sabotaging ourselves and may continue to attract others or situations that are not aligned with our higher good.

Quantum physics enables us to shift the wave to the particle, it is just conditional on which sort of particle we wish to be, which in turn depends on how skilled we are at using the power of thought to establish what we want in life. This explains why each person's view of the world, their perception of reality, is different and unique, we all experience different realities. Known as the 'observer effect', a connection between the observer and the observed exists, so by simply observing something, will influence it. It is not until the observer focuses their attention on something, that it becomes apparent; particles are in a state of potential until they are observed.[9] Therefore, it is in one's best interest to focus one's attention on attaining the highest level of well-being! Although the quantum physics premise that our thoughts determine our reality is not yet accepted in conventional medical circles, this does not stop one from practising this principle. Developing proficiency in creating affirmative, constructive thoughts enables one to enhance one's health or any aspect of one's life. Read about vibrational essences which can help to clear adverse programming and transform negative thought patterns in Chapter 11.

Similar to our physical bodies (elements of which function without us thinking about them), we are on auto pilot when it comes to the realm of thoughts. From birth, we subliminally absorb attitudes, opinions and behavioural patterns from our families or society, and these often become our truth. But we may find ourselves repeating behaviours and beliefs that we did not create and may not necessarily be in our best interests. When we reach maturity, it is to our advantage to examine and question that which could essentially be second-hand beliefs, those which have been part of our unconscious programming. If not, we may be indoctrinated into perceiving ourselves, others and what goes on in our lives, in a certain way, that may not necessarily be valid or helpful. It may be beneficial to ask yourself, *Is my reality created by my beliefs or someone else's? Do my beliefs serve me? Is what I believe and live, my truth?* Barbara Marciniak points out how important this is, 'Your beliefs establish the instructions for how you want to operate your biological being.'[10]

Since everything we create (including our well-being) starts as a 'thought form', we are powerful creators, although most of us do not recognise this. One reason could be that throughout much of our history these abilities have been purposely suppressed by those in authority, resulting in many operating mostly from their emotional natures. Mankind is only just beginning to hone their thoughts and develop their mental bodies to their full capacity, whatever that may be. At this point in our evolution, we are becoming more cognisant as to how we use our thoughts; whether consciously or those that arise from our subconscious, they can affect our well-being and determine the outcome of things that happen to us. One's ability to observe thoughts dispassionately and objectively can be improved by using the technique of Mindfulness.[11]

Developing greater power over our thoughts and elevating them to a more inspirational and productive level, is key at humanity's current stage of development. We are moving into a time (read Chapter 6, 'The Seven Rays of Light') where we are learning to use our minds with precision, think clear, constructive thoughts which when held in concentration have the power to create the results we desire. However, applying effort to our thoughts requires training in thinking accurately. As it is the emotion associated with a thought that gives it power, we need to apply the appropriate energy into ensuring our thoughts are definite, consistent yet energised by emotions which are aligned with our highest good or that of others. Otherwise, one's mental faculties can be developed but there can be a lack of compassion. So, in addition to ensuring our thoughts are controlled, they need to be blended with intuition and centred in our heart, quite often referred to as 'the mind in the heart'. This way our thoughts are more loving and in harmonious balance with heart energy.

Obviously, before we can build quality thought forms that are of the highest integrity, we need to be settled and peaceful in our emotional bodies; whatever we think, whether it be kind or harsh affects the other subtle bodies. We are learning to become conscious creators of matter and that includes our bodies. Referring to his own book, Dr Richard Bartlett writes the following, 'My goal for you in reading this book is that you realize that all situations in life are merely patterns of light and information. If you want to change anything in your life, change the frequency, density, or quality of the light patterns that make up that reality. Let go of all doubt and *do this with a feeling of certainty*.'[12] In Chapter 6, I write about how the Seventh Ray is enhancing our ability to use thoughts consciously.

Consciousness creates our reality or more precisely our own experience of reality which means that mind and consciousness are incredibly important and why it is best we are actively involved in our health, well-being, growth and spiritual development. When we understand ourselves from a higher perspective and change attitudes and behaviours appropriately, our etheric body responds to these new energies, changing itself and the physical body accordingly. Thinking is a great responsibility; thoughts have power, and we need to use them wisely. Mastery over our thoughts (and emotions) and how we create constructive and positive thought forms is not only essential for our health but a prerequisite along our evolutionary journey.

My brain is only a receiver, in the Universe there is a core from which we obtain knowledge, strength and inspiration. I have not penetrated into the secrets of this core, but I know that it exists.
Nikola Tesla[13]

The Soul

We are slowed down sound and light waves, a walking bundle of frequencies tuned into the cosmos. We are souls dressed up in sacred biochemical garments and our bodies are the instruments through which our souls play their music. **Albert Einstein**[1]

Throughout history many have postulated the existence of the soul. If we see human consciousness comprising of more than just a personality (often referred to as the lower nature), the existence of a higher consciousness or Higher Self could be considered that of the soul. Obviously, we cannot be exactly sure what it actually is or if indeed it exists, but from the author's own studies and in the light of any scientific evidence to the contrary, my thoughts on this are as follows.

The soul exists throughout much of our evolution, and it is said to reside on the higher level of the mental plane. It operates as a higher spiritual authority to the lower self (the personality) and is itself a conduit for an even greater spiritual authority. As we go about our everyday lives, whatever happens to us contributes to the soul's aggregate of past life memories, it is the recorder and cataloguer of our experiences. The subtle field in which it dwells is known as the causal body, which has a higher frequency than the other subtle bodies, mentioned in this book. It is thought to pour its nature and wisdom initially into the mental body, then via the etheric body, into the physical. Whereas the mental body is considered the lower concrete mind, the soul is thought to be the higher abstract mind. It is believed to exist on a higher level of the mental plane although it has the ability to be present in all dimensions.

The human body is the means by which the soul experiences life on the physical plane, it can be perceived as a 'vehicle' or 'outer agent' for the soul. We are an expression of the soul's consciousness; the personality is its ambassador on earth and the soul (through the subtle bodies), controls our expression on the physical plane. Our physical body and reality are created by our beliefs past and present and a collection of such collected from previous lifetimes. One purpose of the soul is to complete what needs to be resolved karmically through a physical body and in this sense the physical body is its learning tool. In some situations, it may have the need to express through a body which has a predisposition to ill health, this may be related to karma, and more is written on this subject in Chapter 8.

It is not so much the case that the physical body is in touch with or possesses a soul, but that the soul is in possession of the physical body, it has the upper hand not the personality. Our soul knows what is in our best interests and what is needed for our further growth on the earth plane. The fulfilment of the soul's intentions is paramount in this respect, as demonstrated through life in a physical body. If the personality is receptive, impulses from the Higher Self are received and transferred into 'thought forms', ready for possible action. Richard Gerber M.D. (1954–2007) provides an explanation of how this linkage works, 'An individual's ability to connect with his or her Higher Self is partly a function of specialized energy links within the crystalline network of the physical body. This crystalline network helps to coordinate the energetic structures of the higher subtle bodies with the consciousness of the physical personality.'[2] He continues, 'Subtle perceptual systems such as the chakras have direct input into the right brain through pathways of the crystalline circuitry. This unique bio-crystalline network allows information from the Higher Self to reach the left-brain consciousness of the personality.'[3] A description of this crystalline system is covered in Chapter 5, 'We Are Crystals'.

The soul, however, is limited in its effectiveness to influence the personality, by whether or not, the mind (mental body) allows the soul's intuitive messages to permeate its consciousness. Although the soul is in charge, communicating with the personality can be challenging as the personality, compromised by its level of awareness, puts up barriers so the soul's promptings are often met with resistance. These communications often go unheard or due to the shortcomings of the personality messages received are often interpreted inaccurately. If the personality is trying to call the shots instead of the soul, there is a misalignment, and one is functioning without sufficient wisdom to live one's life fully or healthily. Unless one is receptive and intuitive, our personalities are typically opposed to accepting messages from our souls, yet alone acting on them. It is not until one has developed some level of spiritual wisdom and acceptance of an inner higher authority that one is able to handle these energies. When our mental body becomes more balanced and active it becomes a transmitter of soul energy. However, until this time is reached, and the personality transforms its consciousness away from being totally egotistical and more spiritually aware, the challenge goes on. However, the many fluctuations of life and physical tribulations only serve to contribute to the soul's experience and its own necessity to evolve spiritually. The soul is patient and continuous, whether it is in this lifetime or another, eventually it will be heard.

In contrast to the civilisations of ancient Egypt and Greece, where belief in the Soul was recognised and supported, the actuality that we are souls is not something that has been actively encouraged throughout more recent history. To the contrary, the concept of one's own internal authority has been suppressed in favour of external controlling influences. It is therefore not surprising this connection is a bit rusty! A dis-connect between the soul and the personality is created if negative energies (at an emotional or mental level) block the inflow of higher spiritual energies. The Higher Self sends warning signals to the personality via perhaps a lack of energy, a minor illness, pain or maybe an emotional or psychological disturbance, even a trauma thrown in to get our attention. It is persistent in this, but if these warnings are not heeded or behaviours adjusted in how we live our lives, treat ourselves or others, the soul eventually has no other choice. Typically, it ups the impact to get our attention, establishing, for example, a full-blown illness or dis-ease when there is no other way for it to get its message across.

Barbara Ann Brennan uses the words 'essence' and 'deeper being' to describe the soul in *Light Emerging*. She explains that a distortion in our consciousness (expressed as our intent) can block the expression of our essence flowing freely through all levels of the subtle anatomy into the physical. She believes that dis-ease is an expression of how we have attempted to separate ourselves from our deeper being. This blocked energy, can eventually, over a period of time, compromise the physical body. Suffering (not just on a physical level) originates from an imbalance between who we are as a personality (and all that involves) and a higher frequency version of ourselves (the soul). It might be helpful to continually observe one's well-being status as a sort of barometer, to monitor whether or not we are in alignment with our Higher Self. Our best course of action in every eventuality is to ensure we resonate with this higher frequency — our Higher Self or soul.

The administration of medical treatment for a major illness (the soul has been knocking on the door for a long time and the situation has become serious) may not be entirely sufficient in making a difference unless recognition and resolution of the origin of the illness takes place. If this does not happen, illness is likely to continue to escalate or return at a later date. The unfolding of the soul's wisdom has a direct effect on the well-being of the physical body. If during the course of physical suffering, some sort of soul awakening takes place, then a complete transformation in thinking or behaviour can ensue which may well result in a physical improvement.

In spiritual teachings it is thought a connection between the soul and the personality is always in existence, but this is according to an individual's level of spiritual awareness and evolutionary growth. Whatever the connection, one of our objectives in life should be to be more fulfilled and fuelled by the soul's wisdom. To become more infused with the soul's understanding, we need to become more apt at listening to its whisperings by quietening our minds and heeding and honing our instincts. The soul or Higher Self does not communicate in the form of emotions or sensations but through the true underlying essence of something which is usually communicated through right-brained consciousness in the form of intuition. Tuning into this higher aspect can save suffering, and in some cases lives. The energy of the soul must be able to flow without impediment to support our highest level of well-being. Developing one's awareness enhances the existing link between the personality and the soul, allowing it to become more pronounced or well defined. International spiritual teacher Owen Waters brings clarity to how this works, 'When you enter a higher state of consciousness, life's challenges become transformed. Problems become solved, almost as if by magic. Upon closer examination, you see that there are two ways that this magic happens.'

1. Problem situations are energetically healed by the higher consciousness, or;
2. Solutions are seen and these solutions are energetically created in the superconscious mind.

One of the functions of the superconscious mind or soul is to create new realities as intentional energy fields which will then unfold and manifest in your physical life.'[5]

Penney Peirce, a gifted clairvoyant, empath, counsellor, lecturer and trainer specializing in intuition development is also the author of several books. In *Frequency* she uses the term 'home frequency' to describe our natural soul vibration; this is the way we can choose to feel if we wish. Of course, our personal vibration is affected by other people's vibrations and the vibrations of the world, but how one chooses to feel is in the end, one's own choice. She explains, 'When you choose to attune to the frequency of your soul, your personal vibration stabilizes at your "home frequency".'[6] She continues, 'Your personal vibration or energy state is a blend of the contracted or expended frequencies of your body, emotions, and thoughts at any given moment. The more you allow your soul to shine through you, the higher your personal vibration will be.'[7] But the soul needs to take charge.

Not only is this soul union important in terms of our health, another benefit, gained through the wisdom of the soul gradually infusing itself into the mind and personality, is offered by William Meader in his article 'The Evolution of Consciousness — Two Merge as One'. 'In the deepest sense, this is the most fundamental goal underlying human evolution and its consummation is enlightenment itself.'[8] An appreciation of what we attain spiritually during our life determines the quality of the soul in its ongoing journey and in our future lives. It does make sense to listen to it! Penney Peirce explains, 'At the soul level, there is no fear or blockage — just clear, compassionate *diamond* light....'[9] Referring to the term *soul blockers* as unhealthy feeling habits (and hooks as our reaction to them), Penney continues, 'Every time you reverse one of these hooks or behaviours and substitute a healthy feeling habit, every time you let go of resisting and just *be* with what is, you allow more of the soul's diamond light to energize you.'[10] It is our consciousness that participates in the continuous creation of either health or illness, the choice is ours — our bodies can be the victim of our personalities or the highest expression of our soul's energy. Are you in alignment with your Higher Self?

Begin to see yourself as a soul with a body rather than a body with a soul. **Wayne Dyer**[11]

Endnotes

Etheric body

1. Biontology Arizona. (2022) *Dr Fritz Albert Popp.* Available at https://www.biontologyarizona.com/dr-fritz-albert-popp/ (Accessed: September 2022)
2. Gerber, R. (1996) *Vibrational Medicine. New Mexico: B*ear & Company Publishing, p. 115
3. Meader, W. A. (2004) *Shine Forth: The Soul's Magical Destiny.* California: Source Publications, p. 250
4. Sheldrake, R (2003) The Extended Mind. Available at https://theosophicalsociety.org.uk/Resources/The%20 Extended%20Mind_Rupert%20Sheldrake.pdf (Accessed: September 2022)
5. Bailey, A. A. (2007) *Esoteric Healing.* London: Lucis Press Ltd, p. 73
6. From the book *Path of Empowerment.* Copyright © 2004 by Barbara Marciniak, p.44. Reprinted with permission by New World Library, Novato, CA. www.newworldlibrary. com
7. Parisi, J. (2011) *An Interview with Beverly Rubik, PhD.* Available at https://www.neshealth.jp/report/quantumHealth/ QH14_150.pdf (Accessed: September 2022)
8. Frederick Lenz quote. Available at https://quotefancy. com/quote/1749761/Frederick-Lenz-The-subtle-physical-body-is-made-up-of-strands-of-luminous-energy-and-the (Accessed: September 2022)

Emotional body

1. Buddha quote. Available at https://moralstories26.com/ buddha-quotes-on-self-care-spiritual/#google_vignette (Accessed: September 2022)

2.   Tolle, E. (2001) *The Power of Now.* UK: Hodder and Stoughton

3.   Hawkins, D (2014) *Power vs. Force: The Hidden Determinants of Human Behaviour*, UK: Hay House

4.   The Free Dictionary. A description of Logarithms. Available at https://www.thefreedictionary.com/logarithmic for a description of logarithms (Accessed: September 2022)

5.   Pert, C. (1998) *Molecules of Emotion.* London: Simon & Schuster UK Ltd

6.   Lipton, B. *What is Epigenetics.* Available at http://www.brucelipton.com/what-epigenetics (Accessed: September 2022)

7.   The Minds Journal. Quote by Neale Donald Walsch. Available at http://www.themindsjournal.com/quantum-physics-tell-us-nothing-observed-unaffected-observer/ (Accessed: September 2022)

8.   Bailey, A. A. (2007) *Esoteric Healing.* London: Lucis Press Ltd, p. 625

9.   Rennison, S. J. (2008) *Tuning the Diamonds: Electromagnetism & Spiritual Evolution.* 2nd edition. England: Joyfire Publishing, p. 185

10. HeartMath (2021) For more than 25 years HeartMath have been researching the heart-brain connection and learning how the heart influences our perceptions, emotions, intuition and health. They advocate using a system of simple and powerful self-regulation techniques to transform stress into resilience and to live life with more heart, health and happiness. Available at http://www.heartmath.com (Accessed: September 2022)

11. Barrett, S. (2013) *Secrets of your Cells.* Colorado: Sounds True, Inc, p .65

12. Griscom, C. (1986) *Time Is an Illusion.* USA: Simon Schuster, p. 60

13. Vywamus, (channelled by Janet McClure) (1989) *Scopes of Dimensions.* Arizona: 3 Light Technology Publishing

14. Rennison, S. J. (2008) *Tuning the Diamonds: Electromagnetism & Spiritual Evolution*, 2nd edition. England: Joyfire Publishing, p. 184

15. Triv, L. (2013) *The Human Energy Field: An Interview with Valerie V. Hunt, Ph.D.* Available at http://www.healthontheedge.wordpress.com/2012/01/28/the-human-energy-field-an-interview-with-valerie-v-hunt-ph-d/ (Accessed: September 2022)

16. Buddha quote. Available at https://www.goodreads.com/quotes/6990654-what-you-think-you-become-what-you-feel-you-attract (Accessed: September 2022)

Mental Body

1. Buddha quote. Available at http://www.goodreads.com/quotes/1269-all-that-we-are-is-the-result-of-what-we (Accessed: September 2022)

2. Hodgson, J. (1985) *Astrology: The Sacred Science.* England: The White Eagle Publishing Trust, p. 42

3. Sheldrake, R (2003) *The Extended Mind.* Available at https://theosophicalsociety.org.uk/Resources/The%20Extended%20Mind_Rupert%20Sheldrake.pdf (Accessed: September 2022)

4. McTaggart, L. (2003) *The Field.* UK: Harper Collins Ltd, p.124

   McTaggart, references Laszlo, E. (1995) *Interconnected Universe: Conceptual Foundations of Transdisciplinary Unified Theory.* Singapore: World Scientific

   The Field is not only the name of Lynne's book but used to describe Zero Point Field — an ocean of microscopic vibrations in the space between things, a quantum field where everything is connected.

5. McTaggart, L. (2003) *The Field.* UK: Harper Collins Ltd, p.125

6. Brennan, B. A. (1993) *Light Emerging*. New York: Bantam Books
7. Lipton, B. H. (2005) *The Biology of Belief*. UK: Cygnus Books, p. 169
8. Singer, B. (2019) *The Crystal Blueprint*. UK: Hay House, p. 137
9. Mayeux, J (2020) *Quantum Physics and Consciousness*. Available at https://www.beawake.com/2020/02/04/quantum-physics-and-consciousness/ (Accessed: September 2022)
10. From the book *Path of Empowerment*. Copyright © 2004 by Barbara Marciniak, p.92. Reprinted with permission by New World Library, Novato, CA. www.newworldlibrary.com
11. Mindfulness. Available at https://www.mindful.org (Accessed: September 2022)
12. Bartlett, R. (2009) New York: *The Physics of Miracles*. Atria Books, p. 27
13. Nikola Tesla quote. Available at https://www.quotes.net/quote/64430 (Accessed: September 2022)

The Soul

1. Einstein quote. Available at https://quotefancy.com/quote/764435/Albert-Einstein-We-are-slowed-down-sound-and-light-waves-a-walking-bundle-of-frequencies (Accessed: September 2022)
2. Gerber, R. (1996) V*ibrational Medicine. New Mexico: B*ear & Company Publishing. p. 256
3. Gerber, R. (1996) V*ibrational Medicine. New Mexico: B*ear & Company Publishing. p. 258
4. Brennan, B. A. (1993) *Light Emerging*. New York: Bantam Books
5. Waters, W. (2021) *The Golden Key*. Available at http://www.spiritualdynamics.net/articles/golden-key/ (Accessed: September 2022)
6. Peirce, P. (2009) *Frequency*. New York: Atria Books, p. 46

7. Peirce, P. (2009) *Frequency.* New York: Atria Books, p. 49
8. Meader, W. (2013) *The Evolution of Consciousness — Two Merge as One.* Available at https://meader.org/2013/03/the-evolution-of-consciousness-two-merge-as-one/ (Accessed: September 2022)
9. Peirce, P. (2009) *Frequency.* New York: Atria Books, p. 92
10. Peirce, P. (2009) *Frequency.* New York: Atria Books, p. 93
11. Wayne Dyer quote. Available at http://www.brainyquote.com/quotes/wayne_dyer_163897 (Accessed: September 2022)

Chapter 3

The Body's Energy Network

The human body is a river of intelligence, energy and information that is constantly renewing itself in every second of its existence.
Deepak Chopra[1]

In previous chapters I have described aspects of the subtle anatomy, the important part it plays in our well-being, and how illness is a symptom of underlying imbalanced energies. One's ill health can arise from a distorted perception; thoughts and emotions can create imbalances or blockages in the subtle anatomy which if left unaddressed may manifest as a physical problem. In addition, the disharmony created by toxic emotions can thwart the flow of life force energy in its ability to move freely throughout our entire multi-dimensional system, whereas when energy is able to move unimpeded, this is conducive to good health. Each component of the subtle anatomy functions independently yet coexists and is connected with and affected by the functioning of the other parts. To maintain perfect health, all aspects need to function in complete harmony. Barbara Ann Brennan writes in *Hands of Light* that the vibration in the subtle bodies is transmitted by the laws of harmonic induction and sympathetic resonance in a step-down process to the other subtle bodies. Harmonic induction can be described as that which occurs when one strikes a tuning fork, and another fork in the room sounds. If this process is harmonious, all is well, the physical body is healthy. Barbara believes that health is maintained when the creative force coming from our spiritual reality is directed according to universal or cosmic law but if this link is missing, the process becomes distorted and then acts against this law. This distortion, like an echo, resonates to other levels of the subtle anatomy. Our intricate multi-dimensional energy system is constantly creating, receiving, assimilating, and transmitting energies, and as a result everything within us is constantly changing. The messages of our thoughts and emotions whether of a harmonious or disharmonious nature, are carried throughout our whole being. There is no distinction between the mind, emotions and the body, but how does this process work?

In this chapter, other elements of the subtle anatomy which participate in our well-being and facilitate the communication of energies throughout the physical body are explained. The physical body is powered by invisible distribution lines called meridians and nadis, which carry the life force energy. These channels are thought to be similar but named differently by the Chinese or Ayurveda systems of medicine. They are thought to be the interface between the physical body and its etheric counterparts. Gurudas's definition of meridians is, 'The meridians are passageways for the life force to enter the body. They lie between the etheric and physical bodies and have a direct association with the circulatory and nervous systems.'[3] He continues, 'The meridians are held in place or in position by the mild bioelectrical energy of the neurological system and the circulatory system, creating a mild electromagnetic field (partly because of their richness in iron), carrying the life force between the two systems. This and the polarity between these two systems creates an electromagnetic tunnel through which the life force can travel.'[4] These small threads of energy are the etheric parallel to the intricate nervous system, underlying every nerve in the human body, they help to feed, activate and sustain the physical form and determine the nature and quality of the entire nervous system.

The chakras are perhaps the most well-known aspect of the subtle anatomy, and much is written about them. Therefore, it is not the author's intention to provide great detail as many other publications offer this. However, a description of the subtle anatomy would be incomplete without an explanation of the chakras and their enormous importance to our well-being, so a brief interpretation of the seven main chakras and their characteristics is offered here. What should be emphasised is how these energy centres respond to our emotions and thoughts and are instrumental in creating our physical reality. The concept of the chakras originates from early Hindu teachings, and they are described in Sanskrit as wheels or vortices. Alice Bailey, who refers to the chakras as 'centres' writes extensively about them in her books, describing them as collections of atoms, vibrating at high speed and at varying points of evolution. They are thought to reside in the etheric body, and are situated along the spine, but there are also corresponding chakras existing at each level of the subtle bodies, which are connected to and communicating with each other. The life force and spiritual information (from the cosmos) is channelled into the body through the chakras which act as receivers, assimilators and transmitters of this energy. Their activity can be seen as similar to radio frequencies, but chakras operate in frequencies of consciousness. The activity of the chakras is crucial. The energy they receive is transmuted and radiated throughout the body, but this is dependent on the extent of the unfoldment of each chakra. Their condition can vary from being (ideally) fully awakened, active and receptive to the inflow of energies, to the not so ideal, too slow, sluggish, only partially functioning or totally dormant and unresponsive. They can also become over stimulated. Alice Bailey explains the repercussion of poorly functioning chakras, 'In the case where these centres, through which the inflowing energy from these sources of supply flow, are quiescent, unawakened or only functioning partially or too slowly (as far as their vibratory rhythm is concerned), then you will have a condition of blocking. This will produce congestion in the etheric vehicle, and consequent and subsequent difficulties in the functioning of the physical body.'[5] Referring to ill effects due to the chakras being at various stages of development, she writes, 'Such diseases either arise from within the body itself as the result of inherent (or should I say indigenous) or hereditary tendencies or predispositions, present in the bodily tissue; or they arise as the result of the radiation or the non-radiation of the centres, which work through the nadis....'[6] I suggest her reference to indigenous or hereditary predispositions, is referring to miasms, a type of vibrational patterning passed from generation to generation. These can be thought of as latent, discordant energetic residues or types of pollution, left from a previous lifetime residing in the cellular memory of the body and subtle anatomy system. Read about Miasms in Chapter 9. Referring further to ill health and the importance of a balanced and healthy chakra system, she continues, 'they can also arise as a result of external impacts or contact (such as infectious or contagious diseases and epidemics). These, the subject is unable to resist, owing to the lack of development of his centres'.[7]

Chakras energise the body, or rather they should do if they and other parts of the subtle anatomy are in good working order. The invisible distribution channels distribute Prana throughout the nervous system, and into the blood stream via the chakras and endocrine system. Each chakra is linked with a major spinal nerve ganglia and nerve plexus and corresponds with an endocrine gland. As commonly known, the glands produce and release hormones which are secreted into and circulate throughout the blood system, regulating and controlling human growth and behaviour and affecting every part of our bodies. William Meader explains how the energies of the emotional and mental bodies also inform the physical body (via the chakras). He writes, 'Through the etheric vehicle, all energies must pass, including the energies of thought and emotion. As such, the etheric sheath is responsible for translating all forms of subtle energy into something realized within consciousness or tangibly manifest in the outer world. An individual cannot experience an intuition, thought or feeling without the etheric vehicle acting as an intermediary capable of impressing such vibrations upon the brain and nervous system, as well as the endocrine system.'[8] The chemical processes of the body function as the result of a by-product of other forces acting upon the molecular level. The endocrine system is the physical manifestation and externalisation of the chakras which translate energies into hormones. The glands respond to the awakened or un-awakened condition of the chakras. In *Esoteric Healing*, Alice Bailey explains this, 'The psychological causes are forms of energy, working out through the appropriate centres in the body, and these, in their turn, condition the glandular system. The secretion or hormone, generated under this esoteric stimulation, finds its way into the blood stream, and the result of all this interaction can be either good health, as expressed by sound psychological causes, or poor health, as it expresses the reverse.'[9] The effectiveness of the etheric body to transmit energies is complex and intricate and depends on the awakened or un-awakened condition of the energy centres. Although medical science recognises the endocrine system affects us both physically and psychologically, there is little acceptance in current medicine that it is the associated chakras that are responsible for this process.

Our state of awareness is also represented by the chakras. They reflect decisions we make and how we respond to conditions in our life, so when there are weaknesses present at any level of the chakras (which are representative of the glands/ organs), it is likely to indicate one is having difficulties with the psychological issues and life experiences associated with that chakra. Alice Bailey substantiates this, 'But behind this condition of the glandular system lies the basic imbalance of the centres themselves.'[10] She continues, 'All the subsidiary organs of man are effects; they are not pre-determining causes. The determining causes in man, and that which makes him what he is, are the glands. They are externalisations of the types of force pouring through the etheric centres from the subtler worlds of being. They express the point in evolution which the man has reached; they are vital and active or non-vital and inactive, according to the condition of the centres. They demonstrate a sufficiency, an oversufficiency or a deficiency, according to the condition of the etheric vortices.'[11] Alice Bailey uses the word vortices to describe the spinning, whirlpool nature of the chakras.

My very brief description of the seven main (there are others, not covered in this book) chakras follows, but other cultures (and therefore their texts) may have slightly different interpretations. When a chakra is unbalanced, illness or disharmony related to the corresponding organs may occur. Note, however, that the chakra system is in a process of change as humanity evolves.

The Base chakra is associated with basic raw energy, self-awareness, our survival instincts, and being able to feel grounded and secure. It is linked to the skeleton, the feet, the excretory organs and the adrenals.

The Sacral chakra is linked with pleasure, creativity, courage, assertion, self-respect, self-responsibility and sexual issues. It is related to the reproductive and urinary systems, the pelvis area, lower back, emotional or psychological problems.

The Solar plexus chakra is to do with self-esteem, emotions, instincts, our sense of power and drive. It is also associated with self-worth. It is linked with the stomach, liver, gall bladder, spleen and pancreas. It governs digestive functions, not just physically but our ability to digest and assimilate feelings and experiences.

The Heart chakra is associated with compassion, unconditional love of self and others, and universal goodwill. It is associated with the heart, respiratory organs, upper limbs and the thymus. It governs the circulation and is linked with heart or respiratory problems such as asthma.

The Throat chakra is associated with communication, creativity, and self-expression. It relates to the transition from personal to higher will, and the ability to express oneself authentically. It is linked with the throat, ears, immunity, the thyroid gland, neck and shoulders.

The Brow chakra enables us to connect with the non-physical. It is to do with intuition, imagination and awareness. It is known as the seat of perception, insight, clairvoyance and spiritual sight. It governs cognition, vision and intellect. It is linked with the pituitary gland, hypothalamus, nervous system, and the brain. There is variance here in that many texts associate it with the pineal gland and the crown chakra (see below) with the pituitary gland.

The Crown chakra is the link to our highest source of guidance. It relates to our intuition and links us with the universal life force, our Higher Self and a higher power, whatever we wish to call this. It is the centre through which consciousness functions and through which we connect on a spiritual level, and it is linked with the pineal gland (see above).

During the process of our evolution one of our life tasks is to manage the psychological issues linked to each of the chakras, although it may only be one issue we are addressing in a lifetime. To give an example, if digestive issues are experienced this could point to a solar plexus chakra imbalance and it may be appropriate to work on improving self-esteem. Whenever we experience tension, for example, this is detected by the nerve plexus associated with each chakra and transmitted to the part of the body controlled by that plexus. If we continue, over time, to endure prolonged or intense stress, apart from eventually depleting the immune system, this may manifest as a physical symptom such as discomfort, pain or illness. This is an example of how we create our own reality. We receive a message (symptom) about something in our life which needs addressing and it is for us to interpret that message, interrupt the negative flow of energies by changing the nature of our thoughts, feelings and behaviours and hence our well-being. If we are successful in handling issues related to the chakras, we are not only improving our well-being, but we are bringing each chakra into greater functioning consciousness. The activities and outcomes of our experiences in previous lives are registered with karmic law which is related to the building of the physical body and what constitutes the personality. Alice Bailey writes, 'the karmic process in any individual life must therefore work out through the medium of the glands, which condition the reaction of the person to circumstance and events.'[12]

It is clear from her writings, she considers there are additional factors other than emotions, thoughts, life force energy and karma which can impact the chakras. 'It is a secondary truism that this etheric body is the conveyor of the forces of the personality, through the medium of the centres, and thereby galvanises the physical body into activity. These forces, routed through the centres, are those of the integrated personality as a whole, or are simply the forces of the astral or emotional body and the mind body; they also transmit the force of the personality ray or the energy of the soul ray, according to the point in evolution reached by the man. The physical body, therefore, is not a principle. *It is conditioned and does not condition* — a point oft forgotten.'[13] The personality and soul Rays she mentions are aspects of the 'Seven Rays', which according to ancient tradition, are seven bands of light energy which derive from cosmic sources and pervade and energise our planet and all forms of life on it. Read more about the 'Seven Rays' in Chapter 6. The seven chakras (and our energy fields) are recipients of these Seven Rays, and act as transformers converting their high vibrational energies into a form the physical body can process. The soul and personality Rays determine our potential for strengths and weaknesses, mentally, emotionally, spiritually and physically.

Information of an energetic nature spreads throughout the body through the blood and the nervous system, our bodies are an incredible complex communication network of resonance and frequency.

The next chapter expands on the concept of connectiveness, communication and our connections with others.

The energy of life entering and leaving your body flows evenly throughout the universe. With that current, the mind of the cosmos communicates with all things. **Ilchi Lee**[14]

Endnotes

1. Deepak Chopra quote. Available at https://quotefancy. com/quote/793143/Deepak-Chopra-The-human-body-is-river-of-intelligence-energy-and-information (Accessed: September 2022)

2. Brennan, B. A. (1988) *Hands of Light.* New York: Bantam Books

3. Gurudas. (1985) *Gem Elixirs and Vibrational Healing, Vol. I.* California: Cassandra, p. 56

4. Gurudas. (1985) *Gem Elixirs and Vibrational Healing, Vol. I.* California: Cassandra, p. 56

5. Bailey, A. A. (2007) *Esoteric Healing.* London: Lucis Press Ltd, p. 74

6. Bailey, A. A. (2007) *Esoteric Healing.* London: Lucis Press Ltd, p. 198

7. Bailey, A. A. (2007) *Esoteric Healing.* London: Lucis Press Ltd, p. 198

8. Meader, W. A. (2004) *Shine Forth: The Soul's Magical Destiny.* California: Source Publications, p. 250

9. Bailey, A. A. (2007) *Esoteric Healing.* London: Lucis Press Ltd, p. 337

.

10. Bailey, A. A. (2007) *Esoteric Healing.* London: Lucis Press Ltd, p. 84

Note: centres are another word for chakras.

11. Bailey, A. A. (2007) *Esoteric Healing.* London: Lucis Press Ltd, p. 46

12. Bailey, A. A. (2007) *Esoteric Healing.* London: Lucis Press Ltd, p. 624

13. Bailey, A. A. (2007) *Esoteric Healing.* London: Lucis Press Ltd, p. 190

14. Ilchi Lee quote. Available at https://www.goodreads.com/quotes/tag/energy-healing?page=5 (Accessed: September 2022)

Chapter 4

We Are All One

The new physics provides a modern version of ancient spirituality. In a universe made out of energy, everything is entangled; everything is one. **Bruce H Lipton**[1]

Previous chapters describe elements of our multi-dimensional subtle anatomy and its electromagnetic field emission. Not only are we energy, but we are also surrounded by and exist in a world of infinite energy, everything around us also operates as a frequency. At one time, Space was thought to be empty but is now considered to be full of information. Electromagnetic waves of cosmic radiation conveying vast amounts of information travel through space, their vibrations are constantly working upon us; we receive knowledge from and are in dialogue with the universe. We are enmeshed in a matrix of energetic relationships where we are constantly sending out and receiving information from others and from the cosmos. Alice Bailey endorses this, 'It is through the etheric body that all the energies flow, whether emanating from the soul, or from the sun, or from a planet.'[2] Perhaps it is not surprising that scientists studying subatomic particles and realising they are displaying signs of consciousness, are concluding that the universe and everything in it, must be conscious. The universe appears to be one huge, aware, interconnected, and infinite energetic being!

As we interact with and respond to subtle frequencies and vibrations of the universe, we are instantaneously and constantly 'tuning' ourselves according to the information received. As we exist in a vast field of energy, our mental body enables us, if we are aware, to tap into a multi-dimensional pool of wisdom, providing us with information which can be supportive of the health of our bodies, minds and souls. Since everything is connected, we have the power to access far greater information than most of us are unaware of. Taking radio frequencies again as an analogy, Itzhak Bentov (1923–1979) a scientist, inventor, mystic and author, believes the basic underlying function of our physical and other bodies is to pick up signals or stimuli, process them, and respond to them. He writes, 'Suppose now that we visualise ourselves as a radio-like device that is receiving four or five different stations simultaneously. One station will by far over shadow the others in loudness, and among the others there are also differences in their degree of loudness. We can liken the strongest station to the physical reality. Whatever comes in through this channel is heard most strongly, while the other "stations" representing the astral, mental, causal, and spiritual realities are successively weaker.... The important thing to realize is that we are capable of listening to all stations simultaneously.'[3]

We are not only energetically connected to the Universe but to all other humans, which explains how certain people, with heightened perceptions, are capable of feeling, sensing and picking up subtle influences about others or circumstances without having had a prior logical reason or explanation for them. Since we exist within a vast field of vibrations, it can be difficult to define our boundaries, as we are not separate, we are part of the whole. Our personal vibration impacts others. Everything we think, say, and do affects them, as they do to us, yet many people are totally unaware of the physical effect that others can have on them. Since we are affected by other people's energies, it is vital to reinforce our energetic boundaries and depending on how successful we are at doing this, energies from others may strengthen and support us, or devitalise and debilitate us. The more able we are in establishing healthy boundaries, the greater our ability to manage energy which contributes to our well-being. Learning to transmute negative thoughts received from others into positive ones, is also a valuable skill to learn.

In his book *Wholeness and the Implicate Order*, theoretical physicist Professor David Bohm (1917–1992) conveys the understanding that despite humankind thinking to the contrary, things are not separate and independent of each other. His findings indicate that although we perceive the world in this way, we are actually doing so to make our lives manageable, yet in reality everything and everyone are connected. The implications of his theory supply a much larger picture of a human being in as much as we are not isolated bodies and personalities, we are part of a complex energy matrix which is connected not only to everyone else but to everything else. This concept of 'everyone and everything' can be extended further. Some spiritual philosophies believe that all forms of life are conscious, evolving and contained within a higher pattern or template; we are all part of a great plan of creation. In every living system there exists the understanding 'as above, so below', also known as the Law of Correspondences. What happens in the microcosm also happens in the macrocosm: as an example, what occurs on the spiritual planes also occurs on the earth plane. This law pertains to the understanding that every unit of life lives, moves and has its being within the body of a greater unit of life of which the lesser is a reflection. Similar to our bodies consisting of cells, we too (as humans) are a living body of consciousness which is also part of a higher consciousness. Joan Hodgson writes, 'Although each man is an individual unit with infinite possibilities for development, at the same time he is one with the whole cosmic scheme, even as the cells of a living organism are units and yet parts of the whole.'[4] From an esoteric perspective, planets in our solar system are incarnations of evolving consciousnesses. They are the equivalent to chakras within the body of a higher being whose body is our solar system. Our solar system is a higher being which is within the body of an even higher being, and so on. The word 'higher' could be read here as more advanced in consciousness. As an example, we may contrast the functioning of a single cell within a physical body, to a person living in a community. Using this analogy and from an esoteric perspective, humans are a type of cell or chakra within planet Earth, which is a conscious being in its own right. This planetary higher being can be regarded as what some may call God, but others may prefer alternative terms such as 'Source'. The solar higher being can be seen as a 'god' of an even higher order. In his book, William Meader affirms this, 'Each of us is part of the collective consciousness of humanity as a whole. Indeed, from the esoteric perspective, humanity is considered a single entity within the body of our planetary god.'[5] All principles contained in bodies are contained in the macrocosm, the universe also being within one. It is also a belief of Mahatma Gandhi (1869–1948), the primary leader of India's independence movement and architect of forms of non-violent civil disobedience. He wrote, 'The human body is the universe in miniature. That which cannot be found in the body is not found in the universe. Hence the philosopher's formula, that the universe within reflects the universe without.'[6]

We are intimately connected to everything else; our individual etheric bodies are part of the etheric body of humanity, which is part of the etheric body of the planet, which is part of the etheric body of the solar system, and so on. Humans can be seen as being the microcosm, even at the level of our well-being, for when our whole system, mind, body and spirit are in balance we experience good health.

The consciousness within our solar system is always evolving, so as we evolve so does the earth and all the planets in our solar system including the higher beings. If as a humanity we experience turbulence then so does the higher being, much like (on a lower level) an ingrowing toenail, we are going to know about it! The more harmonious we are mentally, emotionally, physically and spiritually effects not only ourselves and others, but higher consciousnesses, in a beneficial way. This becomes easier as we learn to respond adequately to the subtle impulses from our souls. Words from Alice Bailey remind us just how connected we are. 'It should be remembered that the etheric body of the human being is an integral part of the etheric body of the planetary Logos[7] and is, therefore, related to all forms found within that body in any and all the kingdoms in nature. It is part of the substance of the universe, coordinated with planetary substance, and hence provides the scientific basis for unity.'[8]

Consistent with the description of the subtle anatomy as a hologram (mentioned earlier in this book), the universe has also been described by scientists as holographic by design. Both author Michael Talbot (1953–1992)[9] and Richard Gerber M.D. (1954–2007) suggest the universe itself is a gigantic 'cosmic hologram'. Richard writes, 'By virtue of its likely holographic characteristics, every piece of the universe not only contains but also contributes to the information of the whole.'[10]

Jude Currivan, Ph.D., cosmologist, planetary healer and futurist, is a life-long researcher into the nature of reality and integrates leading-edge science, consciousness and universal wisdom teachings into a holistic whole-world view. She believes that our reality is innately informed and holographically manifested. The Universe exists and evolves as a cosmic hologram, a coherent entity with information its most fundamental substance, more primary than energy, matter, space and time.[11]

The human body is not only a remarkable communication system, but part of a greater reality in which we can experience many different levels of consciousness beyond our normal perception. The next chapter explains more about how this process works.

Just as every portion of a hologram contains the image of the whole, every portion of the universe enfolds the whole.
Every cell in our body enfolds the entire cosmos. **Michael Talbot**[12]

Endnotes

1. Bruce Lipton quote Available at https://quotefancy. com/quote/1519540/Bruce-H-Lipton-The-new-physics-provides-a-modern-version-of-ancient-spirituality-In-a (Accessed: September 2022)
2. Bailey, A. A. (2014) *A Treatise on White Magic.* London: Lucis Press Ltd, p. 105
3. Bentov, I. (1998) *Stalking the Wild Pendulum.* USA: Inner Traditions, p. 113
4. Hodgson, J. (1985) *Astrology the Sacred Science.* England: The White Eagle Publishing Trust, p. 3
5. Meader, W. A. (2004) *Shine Forth: The Soul's Magical Destiny.* California: Source Publications, p. 290
6. Gandhi, M. K. *The Key to Health.* Available at https://www. mkgandhi.org/ebks/key_to_health.pdfKey to Health p.7 (Accessed: September 2022)
7. The word Logos has had various usages but in this context denotes a deity or a principle of creation or emanation.
8. Bailey, A. A. (2007) *Esoteric Healing.* London: Lucis Press Ltd, p. 82
9. Talbot, M. (1991) *The Holographic Universe.* New York: Harper Collins Publishers
10. Gerber, R. (1996) *Vibrational Medicine. New Mexico:* Bear & Company Publishing, p. 56
11. Currivan, J. (2017) *The Cosmic Hologram.* USA: Inner Traditions
12. Michael Talbot quote. Available at https://www.goodreads. com/author/quotes/112838.Michael_Talbot (Accessed: September 2022)

Chapter 5

We Are Crystals

In a crystal we have clear evidence of the existence of a formative life principle, and though we cannot understand the life of a crystal, it is none the less a living being. **Nikola Tesla**[1]

In previous chapters, I have described the components that make us who we are at a subtle level, a remarkable multi-dimensional energy system. I have also explored how we exist in a world of energies. This chapter includes recent research which proposes crystals underlie and provide the means to power our system and also enable us to tune into and respond to information available in the cosmos.

Crystals have a long history of healing due to their ability to focus and transmit subtle energies. In more recent years, they have been used in electronics to amplify wave transmissions, such as in fibre optic cables transmitting large quantities of information over great distances, and as LCDs in television, computer screens and watches. A relatively recent finding and one that is hard to visualise, is that the human body itself actually contains crystals. Studies have already shown that the pineal gland consists of tiny crystals of calcite, but further research has found that crystals in various organs and cells provide the means by which energy and information move instantaneously throughout our bodies. Their presence in our cells is of vital importance in the proper functioning of the body. An article written in the *Journal of Acupuncture and Meridian Studies* states, 'Biologists have shown that the body's connective tissue network has a fluid crystalline composition and appears to be a high-speed, superconductive network for transmitting information throughout the body. For this reason and others, the "living matrix", as this is sometimes called, has been identified as the primary correlative to the Chinese meridian system....'[2]

In 1996, Richard Gerber M.D. (1954–2007) explained (in *Vibrational Medicine*) how science had recently begun to recognize a new class of crystals known as liquid crystals, which have a structure that is partly crystalline and partly fluid. He describes how biology is beginning to understand that many substances and membranes within the physical body appear to function as liquid crystals. He describes the function of these crystals, 'From a subtle-energy perspective, a number of solid and liquid crystalline structures at the physical level are involved in the attunement of subtle energies within the nervous system and the flow of the life-force through the body.'[3] Gurudas expands on this, 'The life force works more through the blood, and the consciousness works more through the brain and the nervous system. These two systems contain quartz like properties and an electromagnetic current.'[4]

In his book *Spiritual Nutrition: Six Foundations for Spiritual Life,* Dr Gabriel Cousens describes the key to understanding the assimilation of energy into our physical structure is through the awareness of our bodies as a series of synchronous, interacting, solid and liquid crystal structures which forms an overall energy pattern for the total body. 'Each organ, gland, nerve system, cell, and protein structure, even the tissue salts in the body, shows a level of organization with some degree of crystalline function.'[5] Much like the internet reflecting our own (future) capacity for telepathic communication, it seems it has taken technology (the use of crystals in TVs etc.) to reflect the metaphysical aspect of our bodies.

The late Marcel Vogel (1917–1991), initially a research scientist working for IBM, became an expert on crystals and found that the structure of the human energy field reveals the same properties (in material form) of crystals. An associate of

Vogel's, Dan Willis, writes the following in relation to using the resonant effect of crystals to balance and restore elements of the body, 'The human body, on an energetic level, is an array of oscillating points that are layered and have a definite symmetry and structure. This crystallinity is apparent on both a subtle and energetic or quantum level as well as the macro level. The bones, tissues, cells, and fluids of the body have a definite crystallinity about them. The structure of the fluids, cells, and tissues of the body tends to become unstructured or incoherent when disease or distress is present.'[6] If the physical body is comprised of liquid crystal systems in the cell membranes, intercellular fluids, fatty tissues, muscular and nervous systems, lymph, blood, etc., the author ponders, (knowing crystals have the power to focus frequencies) could we, when reinforcing positive emotions and mindsets, be activating or programming these liquid crystals? In the *Biology of Belief*, Bruce Lipton likens a computer chip to cells in the human body in that they are both programmable. He writes that the membrane of a cell is a liquid crystal. 'Their fluid crystalline organization allows the membrane to dynamically alter its shape while maintaining its integrity.'[7] 'We are the drivers of our own biology, just as I am the driver of this word processing program. We have the ability to edit the data we enter into our biocomputers, just as surely as I can choose the words I type.'[8]

It appears that due to our liquid crystalline system we can tune into and respond to electromagnetic messages in the environment. On her website *Ritual Goddess*,[9] author Theresa C. Dintino sums up the message from geneticist Dr Mae-Wan Ho's (1941–2017) book *The Rainbow and the Worm*: *The Physics of Organisms*. 'Because of their coherently arranged pattern of atoms, crystals are exquisitely responsive. Now cutting-edge, scientific research is proving that all of life, including human life, is liquid crystals. The liquid crystal state is one between liquid and solid, a "mesophase," which is a *tunable responsive system*. Humans and life are *tunable responsive systems*.'[10] Theresa goes on to explain how liquid crystalline systems respond and tune themselves to electromagnetic messages in the environment because they are *coherent*. The word coherence is used by physicists to describe the ability of quantum particles to be in touch with each other; when separated by space and time they act as a unified whole. Although quantum particles appear to be separated, they can communicate and respond instantaneously to messages and incoming information with no measurable time lapse, due to their coherence. Theresa describes *coherence* as a wholeness, a oneness, a unity, that exists outside the usual limitations of space and time. Dr Ho's perspective appears to confirm our interconnected (to everyone and everything) status. Theresa writes, 'Dr Ho asserts that the phenomenon of coherence exists in organisms at the macrophase level (larger than the quantum, micro realm), as well. This includes humans, animals, plants and planets. Coherence is a biological reality. The bottom line: We are quantum beings. The quantum realm is not disconnected from us, it is not some disembodied realm out there or under there that is fascinating but separate. It is not just a "scientific discovery." It is the actual matrix of our being, of life, of the universe.'[11] Beatriz Singer (author of *The Crystal Blueprint*) emphasises the importance of our health as quantum beings. 'When we are healthy, our crystal blueprint resonates in unity and harmony with the universe.'[12]

Crystals help to power our bodies, they provide an integral internal communication system, but they also have another use. Professor James Oschman, scientist, pioneer and world authority in the exploration of energy of the scientific basis for alternative medicine, sees the body operating much like an antenna. 'Crystalline components of the living matrix act as coherent molecular "antennas", radiating and receiving signals.'[13] Referring to his hypothesis covered in his previous book, he writes, 'It seems to this author (Oschman 2000) that the collagen and mineral arrays of the bone probably serve as the antenna array, while the cellular osteon contains the electronic state circuitry that detects and interprets the information contained in the electromagnetic field.'[14] Oschman considers crystalline arrangements as the rule, not the exception, in living systems.

MaAnna Stephenson formally trained in electronics, acoustics and music, was initiated as a Shamanka,[15] and has lived her life immersed in the relationship between science and intuitive wisdom. Her book *The Sage Age* illustrates models of new thought which are a blending of science with intuitive wisdom. In it she writes that cell membranes are liquid crystal structures, and here she describes another of their functions, 'A single cell in the body is a very small, very short antenna. Because it is so short, the frequency it transceives is very high and loaded with energy. Individually, each cell is either acting as a broadcast antenna and transmitting its status or acting as a receiving antenna to obtain what it needs.'[16] 'Collectively, similar cells transmit their own unique signal. For example, liver cells differ slightly from spleen cells. Individually, each liver cell would transceive its own signal, but collectively, all liver cells transceive as if they are one large antenna operating on the same frequency. This is the basic principle used in acupuncture. In ancient Chinese medicine, the liver is not considered to be just one specific organ located in just one place inside the body, as Western anatomy would describe it. In ancient Chinese medical philosophy, "liver" is considered to be a specific energy, or vibration, radiating within and through the entire body system.'[17]

MaAnna Stephenson continues, 'The human body is a sophisticated, multi-faceted antenna system comprised of a crystalline matrix that is constantly transmitting and receiving (transceiving) all manner of informed energies. The matrix is mainly comprised of two special types of crystals known as piezo and liquid crystals.'[18] Piezo crystals convert mechanical energy into electrical energy and vice versa. They reside in the bones, intestines, teeth, and in the collagen arrays of connective tissue such as ligaments, tendons and cartilage and whenever these physical tissue components are stressed due to activity, the crystals are compressed into a deformed shape. When the stress is released, the crystal rebounds to its natural size with the strength of the field generated being directly proportional to the amount of stress put on the crystal. MaAnna explains, 'The deformation of the crystal shifts its positive and negative charge centers, thus creating an external electric field. This is known as piezoelectricity.'[19]

It is perhaps not surprising that exercise is advocated to keep our bodies healthy as this activates the piezoelectric qualities and moving the body can release physical blocks which are often instrumental in making one aware of underlying emotional hindrances. It is also thought that positioning one's body in certain ritualistic postures, such as those found in Tai Chi and Yoga, aid in transceiving informed energies. MaAnna mentions that the way to tune this antenna is through the repetition of such practices as yoga (known to slow the heart rate), martial arts or even playing an instrument. 'Through sound, this entrains the body and brain activity to come into a synchronous state and begins to properly align the body's antenna system to transceive higher frequencies by inducing a coherent state.'[20] 'These disciplines also involve entrainment, which is mindfulness of breathing and heartbeat rhythms that bring the body and brainwave activity into a synchronous, harmonious state. Entrainment of the crystalline matrix in this way brings the entire being into a state of coherence. In other words, the whole being becomes one big, resonant antenna.'[21] In this context, I previously referred to microscopic crystals in the pineal gland which are also thought to be piezoelectric crystals, and act as transmitters in picking up frequencies from the environment.[22]

Whilst the liquid crystalline system in the body is not the focus of this book, it seems to add credence as to how we operate as energy beings and the basis of how energy is transmitted throughout the physical body. It also appears to be key in how higher energies are received into the body and is thought to be a medium in how vibrational essences work (read Chapter 11, 'Are Energy Treatments the Future?'). In summary, it appears that humans are large antennae for the transmission and reception of many types of energies filtered through their subtle energy bodies.

It is worth recording that water, an essential element in the correct functioning of our bodies, consists of crystals too. Dr Gerald Pollack, University of Washington Professor of bioengineering, and author of *Cells, Gels and the Engines of Life: A New Unifying Approach to Cell Function* and *The Fourth Phase of Water*, has developed a theory of water that has been called revolutionary. He has spent the past decade convincing worldwide audiences that water is not actually a liquid. He believes that structured water (as it is often referred to) is a hexagonal crystalline structure between liquid water and crystal. He presents evidence that shows water is absolutely essential to everything a cell does. 'Structured water does not have the same properties as bulk water. Water is the carrier of the most important molecules of life, like proteins and DNA.... The water in our cells is not like water in a glass. It's actually ordered pretty much like a crystal. Like ice, it excludes particles and solutes as it forms.'[23] Beatriz Singer, referred to earlier, writes, 'It's also believed that crystals can pattern the water within our bodies, as quartz (SiO_2) and water (H_2O) have similar tetrahedral geometries.'[24]

Structured water is also referred to as organized water, hexagonal water, and liquid crystalline water. It is thought that the human body consists of a high percentage of water which is what Dr Mae Wan Ho refers to when she writes, 'The idea of molecules communicating and exchanging energy by electromagnetic resonance fits in perfectly with accumulating evidence that cells and organisms are liquid crystalline, that all the molecules, including especially the 70% of water, are aligned and working coherently together.'[25] The author of *Dancing with Water*, M. J Pangman, writes on her website, 'Much of the water in a healthy human body is in a liquid crystalline/structured state. Many components of the body are also considered to be liquid crystals, including collagen and cell membranes. These tissues work cooperatively with structured water to create an informational network that reaches every cell. It is the liquid crystalline organization of the human body that accounts for the instantaneous transfer of signals and other biological information.'[26] This crystalline-structured liquid seems to operate like a battery which can hold a charge.

It seems significant that not only do our bones, cell salts, fatty tissues, lymphs, red and white blood cells and skin comprise of liquid crystals, but the water content of the body also contains crystals. This leads one to surmise that water, itself is a vibrational medicine (read more about water in Chapter 12 'Are Energy Treatments the Future?'). If so, when our thoughts are of a high vibration, this could be changing the water in our bodies from a disorganised state to the more desirable and healthier state of structured water.

Barbara Marciniak, writes the following, 'Every cell in your body is a multisensory, multifaceted communication device, crystalline in structure, that responds to the modulation of light — another information pathway.'[27] We are influenced by many cosmic events and in recent years particularly, humanity has been exposed to increasingly higher levels of energies and light. The next chapter explores how one aspect of these cosmic energies is affecting us at this time, especially in pushing humanity to raise its vibration.

Quartz crystal is popular for its pyroelectric and piezoelectric properties, by which it can transform mechanical heat or pressure into electromagnetic energy and vice versa.[28]

Endnotes

1. Nikola Tesla quote. Available at https://quotefancy.com/quote/876491/Nikola-Tesla-In-a-crystal-we-have-clear-evidence-of-the-existence-of-a-formative-life (Accessed: September 2022)

2. Brizhik, L, Chiappini, E, Stefanini, P, and Vitiello, G. (2019) Science Direct. Journal of Acupuncture and Meridian Studies. *Modeling Meridians within the Quantum Field Theory.* Available at: ttps://www.sciencedirect.com/science/article/pii/S2005290118300761#! (Accessed: September 2022)

3. Gerber, R. (1996) *Vibrational Medicine. New Mexico:* Bear & Company Publishing, p. 344

4. Gurudas. (1989) *Flower Essences and Vibrational Healing.* California: Cassandra Press, p. 27

5. Cousens, G. (2005) *Spiritual Nutrition: Six Foundations for Spiritual Life.* USA: North Atlantic Books, p.141

6. Marc Vogel quote. Available at http://www.marcelvogel.org/ (Accessed: September 2022)

7. Lipton, B. H. (2005) *The Biology of Belief.* UK: Cygnus Books, p. 90

8. Lipton, B. H. (2005) *The Biology of Belief.* UK: Cygnus Books, p. 94

9. Dinto, T. (2014) *Liquid Crystalline Life.* Available at http://www.ritualgoddess.com/liquid-crystalline-life/ (Accessed: September 2022)

10. Ho, MW. (2008) *The Rainbow and the Worm: The Physics of Organisms.* Singapore: World Scientific Publishing Company

11. Dinto, T. (2014) *Liquid Crystalline Life.* Available at http://www.ritualgoddess.com/liquid-crystalline-life/ (Accessed: September 2022)

12. Singer, B. (2019) *The Crystal Blueprint.* UK: Hay House, p. 168

13. Oschman, J. L. (2000) *Energy Medicine: The Scientific Basis.* California: Harcourt Publishers Ltd, p. 131

14. Oschman, J. L. (2000) *Energy Medicine: The Scientific Basis.* California: Harcourt Publishers Ltd, p. 179

15. A female Shaman.

16. Stephenson, M. (2008) *The Sage Age.* USA: Nightengale Press, p. 45

17. Stephenson, M. (2008) *The Sage Age.* USA: Nightengale Press, p. 45

18. Stephenson, M. (2009) *The Body's Crystal Matrix-Part Two.* Available at http://www.ezinearticles.com/?The-Bodys-Crystal-Matrix---Part-Two&id=1894834 (Accessed: September 2022)

19. Stephenson, M. (2009) *The Body's Crystal Matrix-Part One.* Available at http://ezinearticles.com/?The-Bodys-Crystal-Matrix---Part-One&id=1894829 (Accessed: September 2022)

20. Stephenson, M. (2022) *The Body's Crystal Matrix-Part 2.* Available at https://sageage.net/bodys-crystal-matrix-part-2/ (Accessed: September 2022)

21. Stephenson, M. (2008) *The Sage Age.* USA: Nightengale Press, p. 44

22. Frazier, K. (2019) *Calcite Crystals in the Pineal Gland.* Available at https://www.authorkarenfrazier.com/blog/calcite-crystals-in-the-pineal-gland#/ (Accessed: September 2022)

See also Dr Blackwell (2002) *Bioelectromagnetics 23:488495 (2002). Calcite Microcrystals in the Pineal Gland of the Human Brain First Physical and Chemical Studies.* Available at www.next-up.org/pdf/StudyBioelectromagnetics CalcitePinealGlandHumainBrainDrGrahameBlackwel.pdf page 2 (Accessed: September 2022)

23. Hexagonal Water and Science (2022) *Dr. Gerald Pollack and Structured Water Science* Available at https://www.hexagonalwater.com/jerald_pollack.html (Accessed: September 2022)

24. Singer, B. (2019) *The Crystal Blueprint.* UK: Hay House, p. 166

25. *Ho, MW. (2008) The Rainbow and the Worm*: *The Physics of Organisms.* 3rd edition. Singapore: World Scientific Publishing Company, p. 135

26. Pangman, M.J. Evans, M. (2022) *What is Structured Water.* Available at https://dancingwithwater.com/the-new-science-of-water/what-is-structured-water/ (Accessed: September 2022)

27. From the book *Path of Empowerment.* Copyright © 2004 by Barbara Marciniak, p.94. Reprinted with permission by New World Library, Novato, CA. www.newworldlibrary.com

28. *Quartz Crystal Meanings, Properties and Uses* Available at https://crystalstones.com/quartz-crystal/ *(Accessed November 2022)*

Chapter 6

The Seven Rays of Light

Health is a state of complete harmony of the body, mind and spirit.
When one is free from physical disabilities and mental distractions,
the gates of the soul open. **B.K.S. Iyengar**[1]

Earth is constantly showered with pulsating energies from the cosmos and as explained in Chapter 4, 'We are One', most of us are unaware that we are continually being influenced by these energies. In this chapter, I write about the frequencies that are particularly pertinent in shaping humanity at this point in our history. According to ancient tradition, there are seven bands of light energy which enter our solar system from cosmic sources and pervade and energise our planet and all forms of life on it. These seven bands of electrical phenomena, coloured by a divine intelligence, govern all of creation and condition every life form; there is nothing in the solar system that is not influenced or maintained by these Rays. The Seven Rays have appeared in several religions and esoteric philosophies since 6 BC. The first direct teachings of them originated from Madam Blavatsky (1831–1891), a theosophist, in the late 1800s and were further expanded upon by Alice Bailey in several of the books she wrote between 1919–1949. Djwhal Khul, an ascended being, recognised as one of the Great Masters of wisdom and compassion, transmitted a vast amount of knowledge for both these authors, with the object of furthering the spiritual evolution of our planet.

There are various characteristics to each Ray, such as a unique vibration, quality and colour representation. We comprise many expressions of the Rays in our total makeup and each person is a transmitter of certain Ray energies. They influence us at different levels and stimulate us to act in certain ways, each person making use of the Rays in a different way. As mentioned, there is a Ray influencing both our personality and soul, and there are others affecting different aspects of ourselves, such as our emotional and mental bodies. It is through the chakras that the Rays affect our emotions, personality, behaviour, well-being and the type of experiences, activities and situations we encounter in life. The degree to which we interpret and act on the consciousness held within these Rays is dependent on our awareness and stage of spiritual development. This accounts for individuals displaying different characteristics, varying from the highest, to the lowest degree of expression if the Rays' qualities are misinterpreted by the personality. At their highest manifestation they provide us with a deeper understanding of our soul's purpose on Earth and insight into the work we are here to do in life.

The Rays influence us both on an individual and collective level. As an example, I will begin by providing a brief outline of the Ray which has had the greatest influence on the collective over the last 2,000 years and the Ray which has been gaining in power, is currently influencing humanity and will continue to do so in the future. Rays move and circulate constantly, continually passing in and out of peak manifestation for periods of time, their cycles influence civilisations, cultures and the evolution of humanity. It is believed the Sixth Ray has been in circulation since before the Christian era began, and its energies have dominated and conditioned humanity for centuries. One of the basic functions of this Ray is to make humans sensitive to the spiritual reality lying beyond our earth-bound focus, its energy is very pure, sacred and tender. It is associated with love, intuition and reverence and at its highest vibration it inspires individuals to understand the spiritual principles which underlie all of existence and brings acceptance and unity with our Creator. This Ray instils courage to fight for one's beliefs and a firm adherence and loyalty to one's principles. However, when misdirected this can result in misplaced idealism and a tendency to self-deceive, often leading to fanaticism and fundamentalism. Ideals can be expressed in an ego-based fashion, with blind devotion, misguided loyalty and with an insistence to strongly impose personal beliefs on others. It is understandable to see how a negative interpretation of this Ray has resulted in many religious wars over the last 2,000 years. At its worst misrepresentation it can incite acts of self-sacrifice and martyrdom and lead to the tendency to give one's power away by devoting oneself blindly to a master, guru, cult or group, some of which breed on fear and corrupt spiritual pretext.

According to Alice Bailey, the Sixth Ray started receding in 1625 and the Seventh Ray of Ceremonial Order has been building in power and growing in influence since 1675. For those familiar with the Precession of the Equinoxes, the Sixth Ray is associated with the Age of Pisces. The Seventh Ray, now growing in influence is thought to coincide with, and 'power' the Aquarian age, said to be the age of science and spiritual awakening. This Ray holds the qualities that will influence how we will exist on Earth, as Alice Bailey referred to it over eighty years ago in her books, as the 'New Age'.

When two Rays overlap like this, with one decreasing in energy, the other increasing in strength, this creates a situation where two powerful energies are vying for expression at the same time. As a consequence, with neither Ray firmly anchored on Earth, we are (currently) between two realities which is resulting in a turbulent period in history. Whilst these energies are in contention the world can be divided politically, economically, religiously, and socially. Although we may be in the midst of a very challenging time worldwide, the Seventh Ray, known as the 'Awakener', is bringing a new vibration to our planet, raising the level of humanity's consciousness and poised to take civilisation in an entirely different direction. One of its functions is to ground spirituality on earth, to show how the world is organised according to a set of spiritual principles, and to make visible the relationship between spirit and matter. We will eventually understand that there is only spiritual substance responsible for producing outer tangible forms; all that is below is patterned on that which is above. The Law of Correspondences was mentioned earlier in this context. Joan Hodgson writes, 'Only as man's higher consciousness begins to awaken does he realise the importance of this law. As he becomes more aware of the permeation of matter by spirit, he begins to understand how every cell in his physical body, every manifestation of his feelings and thought in the astral, mental and celestial bodies, vibrates in harmony with the whole universe.'[2] Often referred to as the Ray of Ceremonial Order and White Magic, one of the highest expressions of the Seventh Ray is the trained energy worker who can bring that which is above down to Earth. This ability is often referred to as the art of creative manifestation. Magic in this sense can be defined as a higher understanding of nature and once we comprehend the rules on how this works, we will understand how to manage energy and become magicians! What appears to us to be magic now, will not be considered so in the future.

The Sixth Ray is associated with the tendency to give away one's power, which has been quite evident during this Ray's cycle. In a sense we have been slaves to our beliefs, victims even, and indoctrinated not to trust in ourselves, but an external power. This can be seen from a health perspective where quite often we feel we should be saved by a doctor, surgery or medication. Obviously, there are very good reasons to seek medical help, when necessary, but in many situations we have given away our power (and bodies) rather than be responsible for ourselves. Trusting in our own instincts and perhaps more natural methods may be a better approach. The tendency during the Sixth Ray period was to divide and separate, whether people, nations, races or religions (2,000 years and more of religious wars) and at times impose unnecessary authority, which further created division. It has been obvious not just in elements of society but in our view of the human body and the approach of the health care system which defines parts of the physical body as operating separately. Similarly, treatments administered with no consideration for the body as a whole can result adversely on other parts of the body. Although this Ray is fading out, its legacy is very evident in the world's tumultuous affairs.

The good news is that the Seventh Ray promotes a more holistic view, it is responsive to the etheric body which as discussed earlier orchestrates the building of and maintenance of the physical body. Greater awareness and acceptance of its presence and more understanding of its influence over our well-being will ensue in future years. Alice Bailey writes in her books that in the Seventh Ray period, the practice of psychology and healing, (in all its various aspects — author's words) will include knowledge of the soul. The Seventh Ray promotes the awareness that the soul controls the personality, and it was her understanding that we can expect direct knowledge of the existence of the soul, rather than just a belief in its existence, as has been in the Sixth Ray period. This outcome has the potential to bring about a fusion of the body and soul, a unique attainment for a human being as an integrated personality, where mind, emotions and physical body function as one with the soul. The Seventh Ray holds the possibility for a completely new way of understanding ourselves (such as being outlined in this book) and a pioneering approach to healing. Considering both these factors (soul and etheric body), this bodes well for a more complete future understanding within the medical profession as to what constitutes the basis of our well-being and ultimately the credibility of diagnostic techniques and treatments that work at an energetic basis. Read Chapter

10, 'Solutions' and Chapter 11, 'Are Energy Treatments the Future?'. It is probable that advances such as these will bring about a transformation in the existing medical system especially as this Ray is said to be instrumental in eliminating/ transforming material forms which no longer serve the best interests of humanity. The Seventh Ray and the Aquarian Age are associated with technological advancements and greater awareness of energy which augurs well for innovative medical approaches and healing treatments. This Ray is said to bring order out of chaos and supply the inner discipline, focus, and concentration required in order to influence humanity ultimately to own its own power and create with divine intention, the best possible structures and systems in society. I wrote earlier about the overriding impact of humanity's emotions throughout the last approximately 2,000 years, and this is because the influence of the Sixth Ray expressed its energy through the solar plexus chakra, which is associated with one's self-esteem and will power. This chakra is related to the inclination to react emotionally from the gut without thought or deliberation, bringing about a tendency to digestive problems. The Seventh Ray is said to provide a measure of order in our emotional processes, which will be welcome. As Sixth Ray excessive emotionalism is reducing, the Seventh Ray is increasing our mental faculties. The Seventh Ray supports the concept that thought forms create matter, this includes our bodies. In the future, humanity will become more competent in mastering their thought processes and with practice it will become common place to use thoughts, affirmations, visualisation and invocation to bring about healing and well-being. A good example of using intention in a cooperative way is the subject of Lynne McTaggart's book *The Power of Eight*[3] where she reveals her remarkable findings from decades of researching and experimenting with individuals in small and large groups using intention. What she has found is that when a collective dynamic emerges it can heal lives and change the world for the better.

The Seventh Ray is slowly transitioning mankind to experience another reality. It is urging humanity to enhance their awareness away from a purely third dimensional level where the perception in everything is physical, separate, with no understanding that one's thoughts have power over one's reality, to a fifth dimensional perception. Earlier in this book I wrote about how we perceive things is totally dependent on the level of consciousness we are operating at. Read about Bruce Lipton in the section on the Emotional body in Chapter 2. We can change reality if we perceive it in a different way. An example of fifth dimensional consciousness is when we live with the knowledge that we have the power to influence things that happen to us. The mental body is attuned to the fifth dimension, and when we learn to manage our mental body correctly, we will become proficient at using thought with intention and creating what we wish. It is thought that when we are skilled at this, manifesting what we want will become instantaneous. No doubt, most of us will need to work hard at achieving this! A fifth dimensional consciousness is far more transparent than our existing reality, as we are free from the laws of time and space, there is no distinction between past, present and future, some describe it as 'everything happening at once'. If we have not appreciated already, we will, from this level of consciousness, become aware that we are all connected (read Chapter 4, 'We are all one'). Everyone is on their own path in life, there is no separation or judgement, as everyone is equal. Awakening to the reality that humans extend beyond the third dimensional reality, will also galvanise humanity to fulfil its potential and embrace its spiritual self. We will understand there is a deeper meaning and higher purpose to our experiences on Earth. Such realisations will also be facilitated by the increased use of our intuition; use of this faculty will become the norm and points to an expanded way of living. In order for a higher dimension such as the fifth dimension to be available to us, we need to vibrate in resonance with it, but once we have shifted our consciousness to this higher level, we need to make sure we become established in this consciousness, as it is easy to revert into a lower dimension.

As the Seventh Ray is associated with order, rhythm and ritual, this is likely to bring a welcome emphasis on living in balance and harmony with nature and the cycles of nature (perhaps observing biorhythms), so vital to our well-being. Healing treatments embracing ritual and ceremony are likely to become more common place, so too are sound-based treatments which have been performed by ancient cultures throughout history. Peruvian shamans sing a sacred song known as an Icaros, to their patients to stimulate their natural well-being and health, in addition to using different instruments and rituals for various healing purposes. It is possible that prayer, mantras and chants will also be more accepted as healing tools. The Seventh Ray has a connection with the mineral kingdom and although crystals and gems have always been known throughout history for their healing attributes, greater awareness of their qualities came into mainstream consciousness over fifty years ago. Treatments employing crystals are likely to become more accepted and commonplace. Of interest is that recent research has discovered that crystals exist in a liquid form in the organs, cells and fluids of the human body and play a part in powering the body, facilitating the reception of spiritual energies and integration of vibrational treatments — read Chapter 11, 'Are Energy Treatments the Future?'. Since crystals (in this case those in our bodies) can be programmed, it seems fitting that affirmation and mantras are used for healing.

Chapter 2, 'The Subtle Anatomy', covered the importance of having a healthy etheric body as essential to its ability to receive high quality Prana. Alice Bailey also notes that pranic transmissions are preparing our bodies for Seventh Ray forces; they will be healthier, stronger with more resilience and capacity to absorb these Rays. She also writes that Prana can be restrained by Ray energies, inferring that if one continually expresses the less favourable qualities of a Ray, Prana cannot flow correctly and would not be in one's best interest physically. This statement with regard to Rays also conveys the main message of this book — our thoughts, emotions, patterns and beliefs can determine our well-being. Alice Bailey suggests that the type of illnesses we are likely to acquire is dictated by whichever Rays are influencing our character. 'According to the temperament so will be the types of disease, and the temperament is dependent upon the Ray quality. People on the different Rays are predisposed to certain disorders.'[4] The correlation of Rays associated with a vulnerability to illness is a field very much in its infancy (as is the understanding of the Rays), but Alan Hopking has collated Alice Bailey's writings on this subject.[5] In her books, Alice Bailey mentions that the Seventh Ray has an effect on the circulation system and is connected to the life force. She also writes, 'The Seventh Ray, however, is more susceptible to the problems, difficulties and diseases incident to the blood stream than are any of the other Ray types.'[6] If this is so, then the findings of Bruce Lipton and Dr Pert, that we can adjust the chemistry of the blood by the way we perceive life, are paramount. Alice Bailey writes, 'Medical men in the New Age will eventually know enough to relate these various ray forces to their appropriate centres; hence they will know which type of force is responsible for conditions — good or bad — in any particular area of the body. Someday, when more research and investigation have been undertaken, the science of medicine will be built upon the fact of the vital body and its constituent energies. It will then be discovered that this science will be far simpler and less complicated than present medical service.'[7] Let's hope so!

It is not the objective of this book to provide detail about the seven Ray personality types, but a very brief indication of their nature and their colour representation follows.

First Ray–the energy of Will and Purpose (red). This Ray is responsible for our physical motivation, it provides initiative and energy. When it is prominent in a person's makeup it is evident as a strong driving force and purpose in life. This Ray is marked in someone who has great ability to overcome challenges and problems and accomplish their goals. The shadow side or qualities to overcome are arrogance, pride, selfishness, a desire to control, dominate and manipulate.

Second Ray–the energy of Love Wisdom (blue). This Ray is responsible for our awareness, sensitivity and intuition. Its role is to support every soul in their quest for spiritual enlightenment. Its emphasis is on imbuing peace, love and wisdom and is prominent in teachers, light workers and healers. The shadow side or qualities to overcome are self-pity, undue sensitivity, anxiety, conditional love or the love of being loved oneself.

Third Ray–the energy of Active Intelligence (yellow). This Ray is responsible for our mental faculties and ability to communicate. When it is prominent in a person's makeup it produces an abstract thinker, someone with a clear intellect, and penetrating mind, capable of deep concentration. It brings patience, business skills, and the ability to plan in advance and understand the practical implications of projects and carry them to satisfactory conclusion. The qualities to overcome can be a pre-occupation with detail, being overly intellectual or critical or an overly strong attachment to materialism.

Fourth Ray–the energy of Harmony through Conflict (green). This Ray brings a strong sense of beauty, form, balance and symmetry in all things. It stimulates creativity and is often strong in someone who is an artist. When it is prominent in a person's character, an appreciation of harmony in all things will be upmost. However, in achieving this, one may be required to withstand struggle or conflict until desired aims are achieved or to balance opposing tendencies in order to bring about greater harmony. There can be extreme passions to overcome, and life may consist of highs and lows.

Fifth Ray–the energy of Concrete Knowledge or Science (orange). This Ray brings a keen intellect, analytical ability, attention to detail, ability to undertake research, scientific ability or a love of science or spiritual science/divine order. It is associated with medicine and psychology. The tendency, when this Ray is prominent, is to believe nothing until proven and the qualities to overcome are over assurance, a narrow point of view, being overly intellectual or lacking compassion.

Sixth Ray–the energy of Devotion or Idealism (indigo). This Ray is typified by devotion and single-mindedness which is often attached to an ideal. A religious or spiritual nature is typical when prominent in one's makeup, also one can experience intense personal feelings and/or a burning enthusiasm for one's beliefs or a cause. The negative characteristics of this Ray to overcome are having ideals which result in intolerance, hasty conclusions, a fiery jealousy, hatred and anger. Sixth Ray fanaticism can manifest as bigotry, persecution and prejudice.

Seventh Ray–the energy of Ceremonial Order and White Magic (violet). This Ray is typified by strength and perseverance, when strong this is someone who is diplomatic, disciplined with the ability to organise, administer and create structures in society. This person is self-reliant, organised and focused. The traits to overcome can be superficiality, narrow mindedness and intolerance.

Whilst Rays have an input on our behaviour and hence wellbeing, there are other factors that can also be considered to affect our health, such as miasms and karma, which are addressed in the following chapters. Firstly, I will explore whether 'disease' serves a function, and whether there is an objective to the experience of illness.

Each ray or aspect of the Creator's consciousness can trigger different emotions, actions and experiences within our physical lives. **Natalie Sian Glasson**[8]

Endnotes

1. Iyengar quote. Available at https://quotefancy.com/b-k-s-iyengar-quotes (Accessed: September 2022)

2. Hodgson, J. (1985) *Astrology: The Sacred Science.* England: The White Eagle Publishing Trust, p. 3

3. McTaggart, L. (2017) *The Power of Eight.* UK: Hay House

4. Bailey, A. A. (2003) *The Seven Rays of Life.* London: Lucis Press Ltd, p. 344

5. Hopking, A. (2015) *The Seven Rays in Healing.* Available at http://www.esotericastrologer.org/articles/the-seven-rays-in-healing/ (Accessed: September 2022)

6. Bailey, A. A. (2003) *The Seven Rays of Life.* London: Lucis Press Ltd, p. 344

7. Bailey, A. A. (2003) *The Seven Rays of Life.* London: Lucis Press Ltd, p. 346

8. Glasson, N. S. (2010) *The Twelve Rays of Light.* UK: Derwent Publishing, p.77

Chapter 7

Is There a Reason or Purpose for Illness?

Physicians, when the cause of disease is discovered consider that the cure is discovered. **Cicero**[1]

There are likely to be many reasons why people become ill. Obviously, it goes without saying, if only the energetic level is addressed (which is the main focus of this book) and one has a lifestyle that is destructive or lacking in proper nutrition, the likelihood is that the body will not work correctly or sustain good health. There is no substitute for a diet high in nutrients, vitamins and minerals, and it is extremely important to keep one's body fully hydrated. In today's world we are also impacted by toxins, genetically modified foods, radiation, environmental pollutants, electro-magnetic and geopathic stress producing hazards to our health, but the repercussions of these (or food intolerances) are not within the scope of this book. We may also have to accept that as we get older, body parts naturally deteriorate, but support through supplementation can help in coping with this. Outside of these factors and in understanding the reason for illness from an energetic perspective, it is well to remember that the human body does not run by itself alone and is not the primary cause of ill health. It is the etheric body that gives sense to the activity of the physical body, the physical body cannot by itself create or manifest illness; it is manifested upon and is only capable of expressing reactions or effects (such as pain, disease or illness). It operates as a receiver and is orchestrated by forces that operate non physically; we could say it functions similar to that of an auto pilot.

It may be that one of the major reasons we become sick is when messages from our higher consciousness are ignored and we become out of sync with our true selves. The soul constantly transmits impulses to the personality and if these messages are received, assimilated and acted upon, there is greater chance this will result in harmony, well-being on all levels of our total self. However, if these messages are continually blocked, disharmony is likely to result, eventually impacting the physical body adversely. Unfortunately, humans in general are slow learners. We often need to experience something before we comprehend the meaning and understand the consequences. Therefore, in trying to ensure the personality recognises, accepts and responds to its message, pain (which may be physical or emotional) and illness may be the soul's only avenue of expression. These may be viewed as constructive messages, drawing our notice to something within us that is out of balance and needs our attention. This 'self-balancing system' exists to warn us there is something wrong by placing responsibility on ourselves, and if we are paying attention, we can improve our well-being by responding to these messages and making changes. Messages act as indicators, cautioning us to break free of beliefs that no longer serve our personal development, or perhaps we need to slow down elements of our lives that may not be working as we wish or think they should be. Sometimes we forget or just don't know who we really are (from a higher perspective) or we may not be following what we really desire to do in life, and illness may occur in order to draw our awareness to or remind us of these things. However, not acknowledging or denying an uncomfortable issue is common. It is not easy. We may feel the cost of changing uncomfortable elements of our life is too high and convince ourselves to settle for less. Whatever the feeling, our bodies loyally mirror our beliefs.

Suffering in this context originates from an imbalance between the personality and a higher frequency version of ourselves — the soul, although misery on one level may bring transformation on another, especially the opportunity to connect to who we really are. Until recently, it seems that suffering has been necessary as this has been the only way for the soul to get its message across. Yet, with growing awareness amongst humanity, many people are becoming more apt at distinguishing and acting upon the soul's message, so hopefully this means it will become less necessary to suffer, as time goes by. It would be preferable to view illness as a signal to readdress elements of our life, rather than something that happens to us by chance. It could be said that pain and ill health are teachers and can serve as a productive and useful purpose. Beatriz Singer states, 'In truth, the body is never ill or healthy in and of itself; it simply expresses messages that our authentic selves are attempting to transmit to us.'[2] It is hoped that in the future, sickness will be viewed constructively by humanity and the medical establishment as an opportunity rather than a weakness. The challenge of which can act as a trigger to effect a change, not only physically but ultimately pushing the individual along his/her evolutionary path in order to reach higher levels of awareness and spiritual growth. The condition of one's health, could be said to be an expression of the level of evolution that one has reached, in other words, the state of our consciousness or spiritual awareness can have a bearing physically. This statement is not meant to infer that spiritual advancement will mitigate sickness, or to imply superiority; in fact, it presents greater responsibility towards humanity and oneself. It includes striving to have greater control over one's emotions, to constantly keep one's thoughts uplifted and live in relative peace (regardless of outer circumstances), in addition to serving and helping others. However, what this statement does imply is that it is crucial to develop awareness that we are more than just a physical body, and all that is entailed regarding the impact on our well-being, as explained earlier in this book. The significance of our unfolding consciousness and its link with physical health should not be underestimated and is to be encouraged, indeed, from the author's perspective, it is one of our purposes in life to become aware of this.

The experience of ill health may be a valuable experience for both the personality and the soul but may not necessarily lead to a full physical recovery. Realistically, even with the greatest awareness and appreciation of soul input, not everybody recovers from an illness or survives; it will always be up to the soul if it is time to pass on. This is a unique decision, the reason being that healing only happens when it is in alignment with karmic law. The death of a child or young person is particularly distressing but the reasons for this are part of the individual soul's decision and beyond the understanding of most of us from an earthly perspective. An experience of ill-health can be a salutary lesson, often leading to an improvement in one's behaviour or psychological understanding which in itself may be a contributory factor in the recovery of one's health. For example, one may realise that suppressed anger over a period of years may be instrumental in creating a state of internal imbalance and a subsequent illness. If anger is released (not just superficially but on a deep level), this may be sufficient to restore health. An appreciation of the factors contributing to the illness may be all that is needed for an improvement to transpire. The message has been received, its purpose grasped and acted upon; the soul has been heard; well at least for the time being. There will always be more messages!

We each have very individual journeys in life to follow and illness can be experienced for several reasons. From the author's perspective, the natural order of things on earth is that humans grow and evolve spiritually, throughout a series of lifetimes. To best fulfil this objective, some individuals choose (before birth) to experience ill health or a physical or mental malfunction of some kind. This is often linked within a complex interweaving of family relationships and karmic liabilities. In such circumstances some people choose to undergo illness or disability as part of their soul growth and what they experience and learn may be a valuable lesson and important to their particular path in life. Alternatively, there are others who choose illness so that another person (partner, parent, child etc.) has the opportunity to care and support them, thus serving the carer's karma. This seemingly unselfish behaviour would have been part of a bigger picture, a reciprocal agreement established before incarnation. Viewed from a higher perspective, what appears to be suffering may not necessarily be so, or certainly it may involve more than we can appreciate from our earth-bound perspective. Another interpretation is that throughout our evolution we partake in every sort of experience, condition and situation and it may simply be that we have not had a previous experience of illness or disability which is necessary to our spiritual growth, and now the time has come to fulfil this learning experience. From the soul's standpoint, we may have chosen this route to learn a lesson, to eliminate a character weakness, to test or strengthen our resolve in some way, although we may not consciously recognise it as such on a personality level. Any emotional, mental or spiritual change or transformation, reached through the experience of illness, can lead to progression on a spiritual level (again this may not necessarily be comprehended as such by the personality) or resolution of a karmic obligation. The ups and downs of one's life from the soul's perspective, only serve to enrich its experience.

Although we may not be consciously aware of it, one purpose of illness could be to remind us of the importance of being in the 'now'. Gurudas points out, 'The physical body is a flow of energy in the flow of time-past, present, and future. Existence of disease means the physical body is dwelling out of synchronicity with the time flow, which crystallizes karma. Being in proper synchronicity with time means you are in perfect health.'[3] In other words, if you are dragging emotional baggage along with you in life, it is time to give yourself an emotional de-tox. The cells in our bodies are constantly alert, listening to what we are thinking, feeling, and visualising, and as they interpret these energetic messages, they pass them on to other body systems. It is in your best interests to make sure what your cells hear is positive and not imbued with negative emotions. As mentioned earlier in this book, cells live in the present and their job is to respond to your input.

The following chapters present other considerations which can input into our health status.

Every human being is the author of his own health or disease.
Swami Sivananda Saraswati[4]

Endnotes

1. Cicero quote. Available on https://www.quoteslyfe.com/quote/Physicians-when-the-cause-of-disease-is-846719 (Accessed: September 2022)
   Cicero, a Roman statesman, lawyer, political theorist and philosopher 106 BC. Available on https://en.wikipedia.org/wiki/Cicero (Accessed: September 2022)

2. Singer, B. (2019) *The Crystal Blueprint*. UK: Hay House, p. 128

3. Gurudas. (1989) *Flower Essences and Vibrational Healing*. California: Cassandra Press, p. 29

4. Swami Sivananda Saraswati quote. Available at https://www.goodreads.com/quotes/154497-every-human-being-is-the-author-of-his-own-health (Accessed: September 2022)

Chapter 8

Karma and Its Relationship to Health

Every Action has an Equal and Opposite Reaction. **Sir Isaac Newton**[1]

Many readers will be familiar with the above quote, which applies not just to physics, this is Universal law. Our actions, similar to emotions and thoughts have a lasting legacy and produce ramifications for longer than we think. The consequence of actions undertaken in previous incarnations outlive our physical bodies and leave a trace. The past affects the present whether this is advantageous or not: 'as ye sow, so shall ye reap.' This is known as Karma or the spiritual Law of Cause and Effect. It is based on the premise that we all have lived previous lives[2] and if, during these lives, we have committed harm, we must undertake to correct this for the scales to be rebalanced. Quantum physics also tells us that we are entwined with everything we have ever encountered, highlighting the subject of self-responsibility and karma.

We reincarnate into physical bodies many times and at some stage in our evolution we become accountable for unacceptable past actions, and we must address our karma. Throughout these ongoing lives we experience all sides to life, have a chance to appreciate every viewpoint, encounter every kind of situation and circumstance. During these experiences we may be rich or poor, boss or servant, male or female, different race etc., until we have learnt whatever is necessary for our unique path. This also includes the possibility that karma will manifest in some aspect of our health. Alice Bailey makes this point, 'Karma determines the quality and nature of the physical body.'[3] She refers to the reason behind the manifestation of disease as qualifications of energies transmitted from the subtle to physical body. She writes, 'These "qualifications of force," indicating as they do the karma of the individual, are in the last analysis the major conditioning forces. They indicate the point of development of the individual and the areas of control in his personality. They therefore indicate the state of his karma. This lifts the whole subject of medicine into the psychological field and posits the entire problem of karmic effects and ray types.'[4] Read about the Rays in Chapter 6, 'The Seven Rays of Light'.

Karma is an obligation established in a past life, but we can create karma every minute of the day, not just in past lifetimes. We are continually creating our future. In addition to karma providing us with opportunities to repay debts, it offers us occasions to take certain tests again, learn lessons or work through obstacles, to grow and become stronger in the face of adversity, all of these may have implications on health. Although we are not conscious of it, we choose (before incarnation) to experience karma requiring atonement or resolution, in order to make further progress as a soul. Karma cannot be avoided, but of course previous actions can also create good fortune and happiness and therefore good karma.

Karma expresses most often through our relationships with others. We can repay karma by partaking in certain relationships or taking on life circumstances, some of which may include the experience of illness or disability, a physical weakness or predisposition to a certain illness. These may be the result of an action that was initiated in an earlier life; it is most likely that we have all experienced disability (for whatever reasons) at some stage in our evolution. Looking at this from another angle, there are certain people who have reached a stage in their spiritual development where they have little or no outstanding negative karma and may choose to take on a life with a limiting physical or mental condition, in order to bestow a service to others. This sacrificial behaviour enables those caring for them to learn valuable lessons connected with their own karma, and may aid their soul growth, not to mention adding a few gold stars to the cosmic report card of the one offering this act of kindness.

Karma is neither good nor bad. It is preferable to view it as more of a necessary balancing in order to return one to who one truly is, rather than in terms of some sort of punishment. Mooji's thoughts are as follows, 'God, or Universal Consciousness, manifests as grace which is corrective rather than vindictive, thus encouraging transformation and transcendence of ego and making way for the possibility of complete recognition and absorption in the authentic Self.'[5] It may seem harsh that the results of our previous lives are taken into consideration when determining what happens to us in our current life, but this depends on how karma is viewed. It may be helpful to consider that everything that happens to one is not just chance and by adopting a positive stance on what may appear to be a karmic situation, can be seen as an opportunity for future growth. After many lifetimes we become wiser, our understanding deepens, and we know unconsciously if a karmic pay back situation arises in our lives. When we understand 'what we give out, eventually comes back to us', our responses and deeds become more thoughtful and considered. Any form of unkindness towards others (whatever the circumstances) is no longer an option, we recognise that hurting others, ultimately hurts ourselves. If everyone were to realise this, and take responsibility for their actions, we would be living in a drastically different world. Of course, even though past actions may not have been physically harmful to others, illness and disability may be required as the means to learn something important.

Looking at karma from a different angle, some healers and therapists believe that distortions in the energy bodies can be karmically related to past beliefs. A life experience can be created from belief systems that have been carried over from other lifetimes, which now affect the free flow of emotions. If this is the case, the best thing is to clear these beliefs. Since we are all energetically connected (read Chapter 4, 'We Are All One'), whatever we do to someone, we are also doing to ourselves and karmically this may have physical repercussions. In recognising and ceasing harmful behaviours which may have once been directed towards others is an important step in minimising future karma. The best practice for the way forward is obviously to do no harm to either ourselves or others. When we move beyond unconscious reactions, we are in charge of every thought, feeling and action. We are placed in a position of true self-mastery.

Fortunately, the evolutionary process through which we are now living is pushing humanity to clear its karma. Susan Joy Rennison states this perfectly, 'We have vast amounts of unutilised potential, the basic ingredients are within us, but energy does not flow in a manner that creates empowerment. Our task is to transform energy stuck in old karmic patterns that do not serve us, into new energy patterns that are in line with our highest potential.'[6]

Life will give you whatever experience is most helpful for the evolution of your consciousness. How do you know this is the experience you need? Because this is the experience you are having at the moment. **Eckhart Tolle**[7]

Endnotes

1. Sir Isaac Newton quote. Available at https://www.goodreads.com/quotes/1406158-for-every-action-there-is-an-equal-and-opposite-reaction (Accessed: September 2022)

2. Whilst the concept of spaces is easiest understood as a linear construct, quantum physics tells us that time does not exist. If everything is occurring 'now', readers may wish to consider past lives in terms of parallel lives.

3. Bailey, A. A. (2007) *Esoteric Healing*. London: Lucis Press Ltd, p. 608

4. Bailey, A. A. (2007) *Esoteric Healing*. London: Lucis Press Ltd, p. 275

5. Mooji, 2022, www.mooji.org (Accessed: October 2022)

6. Rennison, S. J. (2008) *Tuning the Diamonds: Electromagnetism & Spiritual Evolution*. 2nd edition. England: Joyfire Publishing, p.110

7. Eckhart Tolle quote. Available at https://www.goodreads. com/quotes/28276-life-will-give-you-whatever-experience-is-most-helpful-for (Accessed: September 2022)

Chapter 9

Miasms

Definition of a miasm.

In homeopathic theory, a general weakness or predisposition to chronic disease that is transmitted down the generational chain.[1]

Previous chapters mention miasms, and my understanding of them follows. The founder of homeopathy, Dr Samuel Hahnemann (1775–1843), spent many years trying to understand why, after successfully treating certain patients, their ailments reoccurred at a later date. After much study and observation, he concluded that there must be some underlying disturbance, which interferes with the vital force (Prana) and produces chronic disease symptoms. He called these disturbances 'miasms'. It is thought that Hahnemann was greatly influenced by the findings of Paracelsus[2] who came to a similar conclusion in that a miasm is a predisposition to various physical illnesses and conditions, or the potential for them to develop. Hahnemann thought they lay at the root cause of all debilitating chronic disease and may be a contributing factor in some acute problems. The term *miasm* has its origins in the Greek word for 'fault' or 'impurity' and a miasm is said to be the vibrational basis of genetically inherited diseases passed from one generation to another. Some miasms are acquired during a lifetime but most are inherited, in which case they are thought to derive from the presence of disease in one's ancestors. This seems quite feasible as past generations may have suffered with certain diseases (take TB, for example) enabling them to pass it on (in an energetic form) to future family members. This energetic 'stain' can exert an effect through several generations as it is passed unknowingly in the DNA, causing minor to severe health problems. A miasm can impede the life force, weaken the body's natural defence mechanism and predispose it to certain types of illnesses. In homeopathy, the thinking is that a miasm can be identified based on the symptoms produced and any disease whatever its external symptoms are, can be found in an underlying miasm or in a combination of miasms. Miasms are certainly not recognised in conventional medicine which is unlikely to acknowledge a non-physical cause of illness.

It is thought that most people are likely to have a least one miasm and some could have several. When present, they can contribute to the susceptibility of various illnesses and diseases of a severe nature, and they can also act as portals for other illnesses to enter the body. Richard Gerber M.D. (1954–2007) concurred that miasms create energetic/physiologic influences which predispose the individual to various types of illnesses. He writes, 'Because they can be transmitted from generation to generation, miasms represent an energetic pathway by which events in the life of a parent can be transmitted to their offspring. Miasms provide an interesting interpretation of the statement: "the sins of the father are inherited by the son."'[3] This may not be so coincidental as suggested, but the soul's decision, as we are said to choose our parents for what they contribute towards our constitution, physical traits and life experiences, including perhaps miasms.

Miasms can lie dormant in the body, maybe skipping a generation until invoked at times of vulnerability such as shock, trauma, illness, stress or old age. After entering the molecular level of the body, they become active and can affect the genetic code allowing various diseases to become established. Gurudas writes, 'They are organized in the subtle bodies, and gradually, through the biomagnetic fields about the physical body, miasms penetrate the molecular level, then the cellular level, and finally the physical body.'[4] He refers to miasms as a crystallized pattern of karma and a lack of light or life force.

The author highlights the importance of the presence of miasms as an energetic basis of illness; a concept which will no doubt receive greater interest in the future. A short description of the miasms, their characteristics and some likely illnesses can be found at the end of this chapter.

It is worthy to note that the homeopathic view of miasms is that they can express in several ways, bringing forth other illnesses which have no bearing or connection to the original illness. This is understandable if we consider parts of the physical body/organs are interconnected rather than them operating separately, which is the view held by the medical profession. Tomislav Budak is not a homeopathic doctor, but a therapist specialising in treating root causes of chronic problems, using psychotherapy and energy work. He makes the following statement, 'An allopathic doctor would then give three different medications to a person suffering from asthma, rheumatoid arthritis, and sinus problems, while a homeopathic doctor would prescribe only one, considering it to be one illness manifesting in three different ways.'[5]

Tomislav made several observations during his research of miasms, 'A miasm regularly behaves as a subtle and well camouflaged conscious being, located within the energy body, which tries to completely control one's life — the perception, behaviour, relations, and goals.'[6] This makes sense in the light that everything has consciousness. Homeopaths, such as Ian Watson believe they are connected to our thoughts and emotions. It appears that if certain feelings originating from the past are suppressed, they can reappear to continue to assert their influence on the present, possibly even predisposing one to a certain way of behaving. Dr Farley Spink (1929–2021) was the Dean of the Institute of Psionic Medicine and contributed a chapter on miasms and toxins in *Psionic Medicine*. In this book he explains a possible outcome of suppressing one's fears. 'Consider the case of a child who has been abused in some way, and who has been unable, or even not allowed, to talk it out — the result in later life may well be arthritis, colitis, or of course depression, anxiety states, and general emotional or mental dysfunction.'[7] He further discusses how dysfunctional states tend to be passed on to others either in the same generation or next generation, creating sick family groups. He writes, 'Nothing is more vitality-depleting than internal suppression of psychological stresses, which leads of course straight into the physical consequences of "Psora."'[8] Psora is explained at the end of the chapter. Negative emotions and beliefs within family members often involve toxic family relationships. Tomislav Budak presents the interesting thought that dissolving a miasm involves retrieving a lost identity as when we are young, we accept a miasm as a precondition of acceptance into a family.[9]

Clearly, we are better without carrying miasms which can debilitate health by predisposing one to dysfunctional states. It is also beneficial to future generations if we are able to clear them from our systems. We learnt in Chapter 2 about Epigenetics in that it is possible by changing our perceptions to change our chemistry. In this vein, Ian Watson sees miasms as growth opportunities. 'One way we can empower ourselves in the treatment of a disease is to embrace it as something which informs us about our lifestyle, tendencies, habit patterns and emotional behavior.'[10]

Whereas miasms are connected with disease and disorder, Gurudas provides another thought-provoking perspective: 'Miasms crystallize mankind's struggle towards spiritual evolution.'[11] He suggests, we should learn the lesson offered by miasms, which is, 'Miasms reflect blockages in conscious growth that man has not yet overcome.'[12]

As it becomes more accepted that we are energy beings, it becomes more important to consider the concept that miasms could be behind many physical illnesses. Whilst we may not be aware that we have miasms ourselves, it is probably crucial to eliminate the possibility of any existence of these latent residue taints by looking behind ailments and exploring associated negative psychologies.

The first three inherited miasms that Hahnemann discovered were the psora, syphilitic and gonorrhoea miasms.

The psora miasm is characterised by depletion, suppression, low energy states and imbalance in the rhythmic functions in body systems. A classic manifestation of its presence is skin problems, hay fever, allergies, bone deformities, joint inflammations, urinary and sinus infections. The typical personality traits of someone carrying this miasm are of someone who is concerned with self-survival, safety and security. Their usual mode of behaviour is one of worry, anxiety, fear, repression, lack and denial in certain areas of life. They are likely to be hypersensitive and/or over reactive.

The syphilitic miasm is characterised by destruction, decay, deformity and distortion of bodily tissues and diseases of the nervous system. The typical personality traits are someone who holds onto familiar ideas or attitudes, finding it difficult to let go and embrace new ideas. There is usually a tendency to a pessimistic view of life which can bring a range of psychological disorders, or depression.

The sycosis (or gonorrhoea miasm) is characterised by an over production of tissues which carries the predisposition to a tendency to growths, deposits, catarrh, heart disease, cancer, sexual and reproductive diseases. This can affect the joints such as in rheumatism or arthritis. Classic physical outcomes may include elimination problems, kidney or gall stones. The typical personality traits are a tendency to be extreme, secretive, suspicious and of an obsessive work nature. The boundaries of these people are often weak, making it difficult for them to draw a line between what is good for them and what is not.

The tuberculosis miasm, initially termed *pseudo psora* by Hahnemann, was a later discovery. It is characterised by over activity of body systems and tissues and can account for respiratory ailments and continually catching colds and flu. It is also linked with allergies, asthma, eczema, circulation problems, migraines and can manifest as arthritis, endocrine problems and mental health issues. The classic personality traits of someone with this miasm are restlessness, dissatisfaction, with a dislike of being restricted. There is often a desire that something is missing in one's life, which is unlikely to be satisfied without looking within oneself.

Thinking has progressed since Hahnemann's time, and other miasms, including the following acquired miasms, have now been identified, but are not necessarily accepted by classical homeopaths, who adhere to Hahnemann's principles. These miasms would appear to develop as a result of one's interaction with environmental causes. They include:

The radiation miasm is associated with the increase in background radiation and is thought to contribute to cancers, allergies, premature ageing, immune deficiencies, reproductive disorders and arthritis.

The petrochemical miasm is associated with the increase in petroleum and chemical products and contributes to leukaemia, skin and lymph cancers, allergies, circulatory and endocrine disorders among others.

The heavy metal miasm is responsible for the build-up of undesirable or excess metals in the body. It can result in allergies, excessive hair loss and fluid retention. The presence of aluminium in the body has been linked with multiple sclerosis and Alzheimer's disease.

Having discussed various scenarios which may contribute to ill health, I move into positive solutions, in the next chapter.

When you change the way you look at things, the things you look at change. **Max Planck**[13]

Endnotes

1. The Free Dictionary. Explanation of a miasm. Available at https://medical-dictionary.thefreedictionary.com/miasm (Accessed: September 2022)
2. A Swiss physician and alchemist (1493–1541)
3. Gerber, R. (1996) *Vibrational Medicine. New Mexico: B*ear & Company Publishing, p. 261
4. Gurudas. (1986) *Gem Elixirs and Vibrational Healing, Vol. II.* California: One 70 Press, p. 83
5. Budak, T. *MIASMS — A New Perspective on the Hereditary Factor.* Available at http://www.tomislavbudak.com/en/articles/advanced/140-miasms-a-new-pespective (Accessed: September 2022)
6. Budak, T. *MIASMS — A New Perspective on the Hereditary Factor.* Available at http://www.tomislavbudak.com/en/articles/advanced/140-miasms-a-new-pespective (Accessed: September 2022)
7. Reyner, J. H, in collaboration with Laurence, G, and Upton, C. (2001) *Psionic Medicine.* UK: The C.W. Daniel Company Limited, p. 98
8. Reyner, J. H, in collaboration with Laurence, G, and Upton, C. (2001) *Psionic Medicine.* UK: The C.W. Daniel Company Limited, p. 99
9. Budak, T. *MIASMS — A New Perspective on the Hereditary Factor.* Available at http://www.tomislavbudak.com/en/articles/advanced/140-miasms-a-new-pespective (Accessed: September 2022)
10. Watson, I. (2009) *The Homeopathic Miasms: A Modern View.* UK: Cutting Edge Publications, p. 13
11. Gurudas. (1986) *Gem Elixirs and Vibrational Healing, Vol. II.* California: One 70 Press, p. 96

12. Gurudas. (1986) *Gem Elixirs and Vibrational Healing, Vol. II.* California: One 70 Press, p. 96

13. Max Planck quote. Available at https://www.goodreads. com/quotes/1246159-when-you-change-the-way-you-look-at-things-the (Accessed: September 2022)

Chapter 10

Solutions for Well-Being and the Way Forward

The day science begins to study non-physical phenomena, it will make more progress in one decade than in all the previous centuries of its existence. Nikola Tesla[1]

Our bodies are projections of our beliefs and expectations; our health potential exists in energetic form. We can influence this by adjusting our thoughts and emotions and the outcome (good or ill health) most likely to manifest, is that to which we concentrate our energies. Furthermore, when our consciousness is unobstructed by discordant emotions and thought patterns, there is nothing to disrupt the flow of energy through the subtle anatomy, hence increasing the likelihood of good health. When one is at peace, one has a greater opportunity to heal.

The current scope of medical diagnosis and treatment is limited in its understanding of what constitutes the human anatomy from a subtle perspective; the future health model will embrace humans as multidimensional energetic beings, living in a world comprising of energy. The effect of this will bring forth major advancements in preventative and curative treatments based on the understanding that a high energy vibration is required in order to heal a lower energy (physical issue) vibration. When components of our subtle energy systems are rebalanced with the correct frequencies, this can transform ill health. However, for the foreseeable future, surgery will continue to be used but ultimately medicine will include the study of the etheric body in regard to the prevention, and diagnosis of illness. We have the technology[2] available to detect illness and disease at the etheric level. The energy field surrounding the body can be photographed and when analysed by someone experienced in this field, can denote irregularities and potential health disorders before they manifest physically. Referring to the energy field, Dr Valerie Hunt writes, 'If disease begins in the field, then health should also begin in the field. The field should be our place of primary diagnosis.'[3]

Discussing her research on bio energy, she notes, 'We can also display the pattern of disease in fractal images so that even doctors who don't have a background in this area will be able to make a more effective diagnosis, including for conditions where the etiology[4] is unknown. We will have the signature pattern of the major diseases.... We'll have those patterns and the signature of the person and eventually we'll be able to show that, if we change the person's signature or electromyographic pattern, we can expect a cure. The disease or dysfunction will go away. This is the future of medicine. When a patient comes in to see his doctor, the first thing that will be done is to record his individual signature. All diagnosis and treatment will start from there. We have to have the energy field of the person. We have to have the energy field of the disease or illness.'[5] During her career Dr Valerie Hunt developed a high frequency device known as the AuraMeter(TM), which is capable of recording electrical energy (the human aura) from the body's surface.

A future health care system will hopefully acknowledge the necessity of a continual, unhindered circulation of life force energy throughout the subtle bodies, meridian and chakra systems, in order to eliminate energetic distortions that may contribute to ill health. The following comment on the chakras was written over nearly eighty years ago, 'The new medical science will be outstandingly built upon the science of the centres, and upon this knowledge all diagnosis and possible cure will be based.'[6]

In an interview, Dr Valerie Hunt discusses evidence of electromagnetic energy, she points out that even the biochemists say that all chemical reactions have to have a catalyst in order to occur which is electromagnetic energy. She goes on to explain, 'When the pattern of the electromagnetism is disturbed in the body, you will get disease and malfunction. And this electromagnetic pattern can be disturbed in a number of ways: genetically, due to the nature of the tissue, although I don't think that's a major factor; experientially, due to lifestyle patterns; or emotionally, which I think is the primary factor. What happens is there is a disturbance that occurs in the electromagnetism of the tissue, which will eventually alter the chemistry. And actually this goes clear to the DNA. I predict we will learn before long that the DNA is reprogrammed by the emotional organization of the energy field. I am not saying this simply. I have had experiences here.'[7] She believes that all healing that takes places in alternative medicine is electromagnetic, whether it's the laying on of hands, Tai Chi, or meditation, even the thought process, or the person's intent or spiritual state, changes the electromagnetic field and does so almost instantaneously. She explains, 'Now if it stays changed and improved, the body heals itself, and the chemistry reorganizes. This biochemical reorganization is the effect that medicine is working upon. Medicine has never, ever cured anything. The body cures itself. Sometimes, in emergency situations, we need the offset of biochemistry, but not as a cure of disease. It never has cured disease, and it never will cure disease. Only if the field changes will there be a true cure.'[8] She gives an example of measuring the energy field of a person who has had cancer but according to chemistry, is in remission. She emphasises that if the person is in remission, biochemically, but still has a cancerous field, there is no remission until that cancerous field goes. Her experience of this situation is that as long as the field does not change, illness will reoccur.

Ultimately a greater understanding will prevail as to how humanity is influenced by a higher spiritual principle and to a large extent, well-being will be dependent on one's ability to listen to and act upon messages from one's own internal source of wisdom, our Higher Self. One way to enable this interaction to flourish and flow without impediment, is to develop the ability (if only for short periods initially) to remove (mentally) ourselves from the everyday world and cultivate a state of internal peace. Over a period of time, this quietens mental chatter and enables greater receptivity to other levels of awareness. Meditation is encouraged and can, with practice, eventually bring more unity between the personality and Higher Self. It would be desirable, as part of any healing treatment, to cultivate this connection with the ultimate intention of maintaining harmony in our complete body system. To facilitate this, it would be advisable to create roles such as spiritual orientated psychologists or spiritual health advisors skilled at teaching others in this approach. Susan Joy Rennison points out, 'When we work with our consciousness at the higher levels, unresolved issues do not have to manifest at the physical level, hence revealing our state of consciousness and areas where we have issues to deal with.'[9]

In discussing the existing physiological, biochemical and behavioural models used in medicine, Dr Valerie Hunt makes it clear that these models are not incorrect, but incomplete and do not describe all of our choices, actions, and perceptions. Rather than trying to fit ourselves into models that do not encompass all we are, she suggests a new model is needed, the model of the human energy field or the human mind, a field of energy that incorporates all behaviours, even to the highest level — the level of the soul. 'The soul is the apex of the field; it holds the memory of everything that has ever occurred to it, including other lifehoods,[10] and is also the source of intuition, insight, and creativity, and the source of mystical experiences.'[11]

As a new health model evolves, a greater sense of self-responsibility for our own health will emerge and not what today is effectively a victim consciousness toward illness. It is worthy to note that victimhood is characteristic behaviour of the outgoing Sixth Ray, where the tendency has been to relinquish power to a (perceived) higher outer authority. Many of us have been victims in a sense that we are not sufficiently knowledgeable or empowered to be able to help ourselves other than on a physical level. We can suffer unnecessarily because we are unaware that we are more than just a physical body. This results in placing our bodies in the hands of the medical profession who are themselves limited in their awareness. There are obviously good reasons why at times, it is necessary to seek medical advice and undoubtedly many of us are grateful for medical intervention at certain points in our lives. However, current expectation is that medical intervention, or a pharmaceutical drug, will fix one's problems. There are several factors here. Generally speaking, current medical practice lacks an appreciation of the innate intelligence of the human body. Most often, the approach is one of employing outside involvement (in the form of drugs, surgery etc.), whereas, in many circumstances, a more holistic or energetic approach may well suffice. We do not realise our power as creators, and can often, when appropriate, improve our well-being and generate good health without outside involvement. We are raised in an allopathic culture which instils within us the belief that illness and disease are things that we play no part in creating and that they should be destroyed or removed from us, usually by another person. Ian Watson[12] explains the importance of looking beyond this in order to appreciate that our beliefs, attitudes, feelings and lifestyle are likely to be issues behind this and what needs to be cured first, rather than the illness. Although the patient is currently considered in the process of treatment/ healing, there is more chance to heal fully if they participate in the process. Caroline Myss writes, 'When a person is passive — with an attitude of "just do it to me" — he does not fully heal;

he may recover, but he may never deal fully with the source of his illness.'[13]

Quantum physics tells us that our thoughts and beliefs influence the quantum reality, in other words the material world (this includes ourselves). Yet it appears puzzling this is not more generally recognised as applicable to the workings of the human body. We do know from PNI (read Chapter 2) that there are distinct correlations between illness and one's emotions, so if we become stuck in a continuously reinforced negative belief system, this is unhelpful and can be physically debilitating. Although currently there is some acceptance in the medical profession that stress and depression may have a physical effect, emotions are not generally accepted as having a relevance to our well-being, neither have they been generally recognised as having a chemical repercussion, as proved by Dr Pert. Hopefully, this situation will progress in the future through improved communications between science and the medical profession plus education of the general public as to the interrelationship between the body, mind and emotions and the powerful part they play in determining health. Dr Pert's work and in more recent years, people like Bruce Lipton, are bringing about a shift in thinking which paves the way for seeking solutions that are energetic, rather than chemically based. We are advised to be mindful of how powerful our thoughts and emotions are, not just in personal therapeutic application, but also the repercussions of such. Thus, everyone is ultimately responsible for the consequences of their thoughts. This is karmic law.

In order to gain mastery over our emotions so they don't unconsciously influence us in an adverse manner and/or perpetuate a possible victim consciousness, it is crucial how we deal with situations (especially difficult ones) that happen in our lives. Whilst not minimising some people's experiences, it makes sense that how we perceive an event and manage the subsequent repercussions is key, not necessarily the actual event itself. If one is encouraged whilst growing up to see life's barriers and setbacks as challenges to be conquered, then we approach life with a mindset that enables us to cope whenever adversities come along. If we have not had this positive childhood experience, we can be ill equipped to respond to difficulties, which, for the most part seem an inevitable part of life. If we interpret an event as shattering and destroying (whether it is or not) this often leads to a fixed mindset and an inability to cope, which impacts our ability to take opportunities or partake in life with joy. Sometimes life events are indeed life shattering. For example, if we have suffered trauma or loss or been subject to parenting that is abusive, neglectful or wounding in some way, then this can have a huge detrimental effect on us as adults, determining (if we are not careful) what we think of ourselves and what we are capable of achieving in life. This parental behaviour, although totally unacceptable and perceived outwardly as unfair, may have complex karmic reasoning behind it. The ramifications of such cannot be underestimated, for, as children we place our trust in our parents. However harsh life events may have been, it is imperative that we do not permit circumstances or the behaviours of others to influence us unduly or define who we are or what we are capable of. Bruce Lipton's maxim, is 'perception controls biology'. We have a choice, dependent on how we perceive something determines how we respond to life, in our actions with others and in whatever happens to us physically. Indeed, this may be one of our life's purposes; to rise above damaging conditioning in the best way we are able and not allow it to destroy us. Our bodies are holographic projections of our consciousness, we are what we believe ourselves to be, so it is crucial we impress our thoughts and emotions with positivity. In her experiments, Dr Valerie Hunt observed that the more dynamic and changeable a person's energy field, the better it was for them as they are not stuck with just one way of managing their life. 'They can play it in all kinds of ways. Under new situations, emotional or physical, they can adjust the electromagnetic field so that they can cope, they can handle, and they can desirably work in the electromagnetic milieu of the world.'[14]

Sadly, many people experience great tragedy in their lives, the repercussions of which cannot be underestimated. When one is knocked off balance in this way, it takes great courage to pull oneself together, integrate back into life and function with optimism again. Professional help in these situations is, unfortunately not always available, but essential. We all deal with things that happen to us differently and some people are better than others at overcoming misfortune, but this is what life not only seems to demand but is advisable from the perspective of our health. If we can elevate our thinking, see the good in our lives the best we can, no matter what the circumstances, this sends an affirmative message to our multi-dimensional self. There are many personal development books available which advocate reframing how we see past events, avoiding negativity and keeping thoughts positive in order to constructively impact our well-being.

One of the most sensible solutions for our future health is to prevent, if possible, illness occurring, rather than resorting to medical intervention or relying on harmful drugs. A better way of dealing with damaging events going forward is to provide support to people undergoing adversities, traumas or upsets as soon as possible after they occur, rather than enabling distress to foster future potential illness. If attention and support are available in the early stages for these situations this could reduce an accumulation of crises building up in the emotional and mental bodies, creating imbalance and ultimately putting demands on the medical establishment to resolve problems. It is no coincidence that major illness often arises several months or a few years after a person has experienced an emotional shock, loss or set back. Not only should we be attentive to our interpretation of life-challenging events and subsequent emotional attitudes, pre-empting, if possible, illness from occurring, but healing our emotions can also be viewed as an act of responsibility. Healing our past can have wider implications than just for ourselves and our current circumstances — we heal our bloodline so future generations are not affected by our emotional baggage. Working on ourselves or perhaps with the assistance of a spiritual advisor or therapist to help resolve harmful thoughts and emotions, will also make us more capable of being better parents. Hence, ensuring our children's programming is happy, and they are brought up well-adjusted, balanced and secure. There is also an energetic benefit to clearing our emotional baggage, as seen in the previous chapter on miasms. It is thought that these underlying energies, passed from previous generations, contribute to our susceptibility to various illnesses. However, they appear to go unrecognised by the medical establishment as having a connection to ill health. This is further complicated due to their non-physical nature and hence inability to be measured with traditional laboratory testing. If we are subject to traumas or just through the ageing process, our vitality weakens creating greater potential for miasms to penetrate the physical body. Miasms are addressed in Chapter 9.

As previously explained, the etheric body is a replica of the physical body and illness and disease begin in this body rather than of a physical cause. Doctors currently focus on alleviating physical symptoms rather than the actual cause, which is not outwardly obvious. This is a quick fix solution and means that healing the physical body alone is only repairing secondary damage and is unlikely to affect the primary cause. If only the physical level is addressed, this is likely to suppress the original cause of illness. Caroline Myss explains, 'Healing and curing are not the same thing. A "cure" occurs when one has successfully controlled or abated the physical progression of an illness. Curing a physical illness, however, does not necessarily mean that the emotional and psychological stresses that were a part of the illness were also alleviated. In this case it is highly possible, and often probable, that an illness will recur.'[15] This was very much the theory of Dr Edward Bach (1886–1936) a Doctor, Bacteriologist, Flower Essence producer and spiritual writer. He states, 'The main reason for the failure of the modern medical science is that it is dealing with results and not causes.'[16] and, 'So, generally speaking, is the situation in medicine today; nothing more than the patching up of those attacked and the burying of those who are slain, without a thought being given to the real stronghold.'[17] His observations were written ninety years ago, and nothing much seems to have changed!

Any disturbed energetic signatures in the subtle anatomy (responsible for the original illness) can remain with the potential to be reactivated at a later date in the form of the original illness or a related disease, because the root of the problem was not dealt with initially or sufficiently. This explains why some individuals may recover from an illness or are told they are cured, only to experience a relapse in the future. The only solution in avoiding a more serious consequence is to completely eliminate the root of a disease from the blueprint (etheric body). Referring to outer symptoms, such as congestion in the lungs, Alice Bailey writes, 'though it may be exoterically traced to certain and definite physical causes — it is in reality those causes, plus an inner condition of etheric congestion. It is the bringing together of the outer apparent cause and the inner true cause which is responsible for the outbreak of the trouble.'[18]

Allopathic medicine treats everyone as if they all have the same constitution, yet as we have seen throughout this book, this theory is based on a very simplistic view of a human, in reality we are far more complex, and treatments should be tailored to one's total constitution. The same emotional issue such as anxiety in one person may manifest for different reasons and produce different symptoms than in another. This leads on to a need to develop proficiency in perceiving what is behind a problem and to match treatments with the disposition of the patient. Of course, we can help ourselves to a certain extent by recognising harmful emotions and applying our own treatment, such as changing our mindset, reframing past emotions and reinforcing more positive thinking. It is hoped that we will be slowly moving away from physically treating the body with interventions that don't fully address the total problem (and can be harmful) to using the power of our minds or forms of treatments that work at an energetic level, to affect physical changes. Alice Bailey states, 'The use of the mind will be regarded, above everything else, as a factor of major importance; the mind will be seen as the prime influence as regards the centres, for people will be taught to work on centres through mental power and thus produce a right reaction from the endocrine system. This will necessarily involve the right directing of thought to a centre, or the withdrawal of attention from a centre, with consequent effect upon the glandular system. This will all be based upon the occult law that, "Energy follows thought."'[19]

We have progressed to a point where surgeons are proficient in performing surgery of a lifesaving or life-changing nature and without doubt many people are indebted to them for this. However, if we are more aware of the repercussions that surgery can have on us, we may think more carefully about invasive operations or procedures in respect to the subtle anatomy and the ethereal counterpart of the nervous system. Although there has been little research into this area, it is inevitable that our subtle anatomy undergoes some sort of modification or trauma, much like shock which is discussed in Chapter 11. Whilst some operations are obviously necessary, it does bring thought to the wisdom of non-essential surgery. Perhaps one day hopefully we will take as much care and consideration of the state of our subtle anatomy as we do of the aesthetics of the human body.

The cycle which humanity is now experiencing is nudging them to take greater accountability for their own well-being and one of the primary ways of doing so is by keeping one's vibration high. When there is greater acceptance among humanity that we are energy beings, each with our own unique frequency, there will be more emphasis on the necessity to monitor and upgrade our energy bodies, hence raising our vibration. To an extent, this happens naturally when one moves beyond negative, harmful behaviours and emotions, and overcomes false beliefs. Thinking of oneself as an energy being and not letting other people's low vibration impact adversely or drag one down, is crucial. It also helps if we spend quiet time in meditation, self-reflection or contemplation. Gratitude is suggested by Penney Peirce as another way to raise one's vibration, 'Let the feeling of gratitude intensify. What amazing gifts you have been given! Let the feeling intensify even more until it reaches near-ecstasy, until you feel that you cannot contain it. Let it overflow and pour out through your personal field. Stay with it and be in it. Stay focused on your heart. Let it continue to intensify and brighten. You're establishing a harmonic pattern that resonates to the frequency of accelerated evolution. Doing this often will raise your personal vibration immeasurably.'[20] Another way to raise one's frequency, is to use energy treatments (as explained in Chapter 11) to resolve emotional imbalances and mental issues. Penney writes the following, 'Your frequency rises to its innately high level when you clear away your mental and emotional clutter and stop blocking it. When there is nothing in the way, the clarity and warmth of your soul shine through effortlessly.'[21] Managing your frequency not only improves well-being, but it is also important in order to live your life fully and create whatever you want in life.

The more you increase your spiritual awareness, the more you elevate your personal vibration; the higher your vibration is, the healthier it is for you. Referring to the method of treating individuals in past cultures, Gurudas states, 'People were not examined for their particular disease or disorder but for their progressed levels of consciousness. Historically, it was considered the causal format that consciousness was the critical issue rather than as though the healing of a physical disease was of key importance.'[22] Perhaps elevating one's consciousness will eventually be considered an empowering treatment used to help one find their way back to true health. An understanding of how we can be accountable for our own health in this way would mean less reliance on a medical system, but we are quite a few years away from this!

A careful physician… before he attempts to administer a remedy to his patient, must investigate not only the malady of the man he wishes to cure, but also his habits when in health, and his physical constitution. Cicero[23]

Endnotes

1. Nikola Tesla quote. Available at https://www.goodreads.com/quotes/139502-the-day-science-begins-to-study-non-physical-phenomena-it-will (Accessed: September 2022)

2. Many readers will be familiar with Kirlian photography which was pioneered by Semyon and Valentina Kirlian, two Ukrainian researchers, who accidently discovered it in 1939. Harry Oldfield who has researched Kirlian photography for many years has now developed PiP (Polycontrast Interference Photography) in the 1980s which appears to have the same or better accuracy for capturing the pattern of energy on and off the body.

3. Fresmag. *Stewart Dawes speaks to Dr. Valerie Hunt about human vibrations.* Available at http://www.freshmag.com. au/human-vibrations-science/ (Accessed: September 2022)

4. Etiology is the study of the causes of disease.

5. Awaken. *The Human Energy Field: Dr. Valerie Hunt Interview (Part 2).* Available at https://awaken.com/2021/11/the-human-energy-field-dr-valerie-hunt-interview-part-2/ (Accessed: September 2022)

6. Bailey, A. A. (2007) *Esoteric Healing.* London: Lucis Press Ltd, p. 77

7. Awaken. *The Human Energy Field: Dr. Valerie Hunt Interview (Part 1). Available at* https://awaken.com/2021/11/the-human-energy-field-dr-valerie-hunt-interview-part-1/ *(Accessed: September 2022)*

8. Triv, L. *The Human Energy Field: An Interview with Valerie V. Hunt, Ph.D.* Available at http://www.healthontheedge. wordpress.com/2012/01/28/the-human-energy-field-an-interview-with-valerie-v-hunt-ph-d/ (Accessed: September 2022)

9. Rennison, S. J. (2008) *Tuning the Diamonds: Electromagnetism & Spiritual Evolution.* 2nd edition. England: Joyfire Publishing, p. 185

10. Dr Hunt uses the term Lifehood to refer to the physical existence of a past life, a time-space construct which has no time reference and of which the Soul is part of.

11. Triv, L. *The Human Energy Field: An Interview with Valerie V. Hunt, Ph.D.* Available at http://www.healthontheedge. wordpress.com/2012/01/28/the-human-energy-field-an-interview-with-valerie-v-hunt-ph-d/ (Accessed: September 2022)

12. Watson, I. (2009) *The Homeopathic Miasms A Modern View.* UK: Cutting Edge Publications

13. Myss, C. (1997) *Anatomy of the Spirit.* New York: Bantam, p. 48

14. Triv, L. *The Human Energy Field: An Interview with Valerie V. Hunt, Ph.D.* Available at https:/healthontheedge. wordpress.com/2012/01/28/the-human-energy-field-an-interview-with-valerie-v-hunt-ph-d/ (Accessed: September 2022)

15. Myss, C. (1997) *Anatomy of the Spirit.* New York: Bantam, p. 47

16. Bach, E. *Heal Thyself.* Available at https://www.bachflowerlearning.com/books/heal-thyself-ebook-version/ p. 6 (Accessed: September 2022)

17. Bach, E. *Heal Thyself.* Available at https://www.bachflowerlearning.com/books/heal-thyself-ebook-version/ p. 6 (Accessed: September 2022)

18. Bailey, A. A. (2007) *Esoteric Healing.* London: Lucis Press Ltd, p.74

19. Bailey, A. A. (2007) *Esoteric Healing.* London: Lucis Press Ltd, p. 219

20. Peirce, P. (2009) *Frequency.* New York: Atria Books, p. 246

21. Peirce, P. (2009) *Frequency.* New York: Atria Books, p. 91

22. Gurudas. (1986) *Gem Elixirs and Vibrational Healing, Vol. II.* California: One 70 Press, p. 95

23. Cicero quote. Available at https://libquotes.com/cicero/quote/lbc9e6w (Accessed: September 2022)

Chapter 11

Are Energy Treatments the Future?

Future medicine will be the medicine of frequencies. **Albert Einstein**[1]

As explained earlier the cause of illness is most often due to energetic blockages and distortions at different dimensional levels of our total being. Since we are energy beings, and illness exists as a slow frequency, it makes sense to use high frequency treatments to prevent and remedy imbalances. The highest frequency always triumphs. This was understood in past civilizations where sound, light, colour and crystals were routinely used to heal. Unfortunately, healing technologies such as that developed by Royal Rife (1888–1971) in the 1930s, were not always well received. He was a gifted scientist, known for designing a healing device using only electromagnetic frequencies to target and destroy viruses, bacteria, parasites and other dangerous disease organisms. The success he had in using frequencies to heal illness should have completely changed the medical industry, but this information was suppressed.[2] His technology is now becoming more recognised and accepted, as is that of Nikola Tesla (1856–1943), another person whose technologies were stifled[3] but are now being used again and are informing future healing devices. Hopefully we are moving into a different culture that is not dominated by pharmaceuticals. and we can expect a resurgence of these frequency treatments. Sound as a therapy is already well established and listening to music created using the Solfeggio[4] scale, said to reduce emotional and physical ills and transform well-being, is recommended as a self-help treatment. An example of using sound in current mainstream medicine, is in the use of ultra-sound to break up kidney stones.

The medical profession already recognises the vibrational aspect of disorders as in the use of electrocardiograms (the rhythms of heart vibrations) or electroencephalograms (EEGs) to check altered brain emanations found in conditions such as epilepsy or in brain tumours. Although the principle that unhealthy organs give off disturbed emanations is accepted, there appears to be no comprehension that another disturbed frequency was responsible for this originally.

The author's experience of energy treatments is that of practising flower and vibrational essence therapy, a simple, natural and holistic way of improving and transforming detrimental thought patterns and unhelpful emotions. Vibrational essences are understood to have been used in ancient cultures, also by the Aborigines. In more recent times they were rediscovered by Dr Edward Bach in the 1930s when he produced his range of essences: the Bach Flower Remedies.

Vibrational essences are liquid solutions containing the energetic imprint of flowers and plants and are generally taken orally, although they can be used in other ways. The reasons for using essences are many and varied, a few examples follow. In general, they are facilitators, transforming dysfunctional or troubled emotions, mental attitudes, and other psychological imbalances which may undermine our well-being. Their ability to transmute negative beliefs liberates one from being stuck in a damaging mindset which can restrict one's ability to progress in life. They can help the release of traumas, upsetting emotions and unsupportive deeply held feelings. This not only results in an improved opinion of oneself but can also increase awareness and motivation regards what one is capable of doing or achieving. Used to expand awareness, increase flexibility and acceptance of change enables awareness of things about oneself and life, that one was not necessarily conscious of. If essences are used to release fixed or judgemental attitudes, this supports the establishment of healthier relationships between others. Essences can also be used to address various self-imposed limitations which can block or thwart one's ability to move forward in life. For example, when they are used to allay fears, this leaves one more able to take advantage of opportunities and become more self-empowered. Vibrational essences are key in helping to change our perception about things we believe (at an unconscious level) to be true but are not, such as feelings of inferiority. This belief is disabling and restricting but improvements in confidence and self-assurance can follow after taking appropriate essences. Although vibrational essences subtly change an individual's consciousness, they never change who they are at heart. On the contrary, they bring one back to one's true self which may have been rocked, jaded or suppressed by life events. They enable one to take advantage of one's innate abilities, reach one's promise and operate from one's highest potential. Their ability to establish positive feelings and sustain one through the ups and downs and challenges in life are most welcome. Their support makes it easier to negotiate one's life path and overcome any obstacles that may occur.

Traditionally the Sun method is used to make a flower essence, although Dr Bach used a boiling method for some of his essences. Using flowers at peak bloom and when the Sun is at its highest power, fresh blossoms are added to a bowl of (usually) spring water and left in the sunshine for several hours during which time the energetic qualities of the flower are transferred into the water. The water is of great importance as it holds the energetic pattern of the flower. The resultant essence, is bottled with more spring water together with a small amount of alcohol, usually brandy or vodka, to act as a preservative. To provide additional bottles, dilutions are made from this solution (known as the Mother Essence), without losing the potency. Although many contemporary essence producers still use this traditional procedure, essences are now created from many sources using different techniques including using human intention to attune to the energies of a flower without cutting the stem or putting it in water. This is known as a process of attunement and is also used to create essences made from the energy of animals or sacred places. Since Bach's time, many vibrational essences have been created from all over the world, using not only flowers and plants but crystals, gems, sound, trees, sea creatures, and those mentioned above. No harm comes to these in the process of making an essence.

Writing in *Bach Flower Remedies: Form and Function*, Julian Barnard, recognising the presence of a light body around plants and flowers, states, 'This is the presence of the light body which interpenetrates the physical. It exists around all living forms in varying degrees: rocks, plants, animals, people. When an essence is prepared this light body is released into spring water, the resonance transfer, which gives a particular quality to the essence.'[5] He goes on to write, 'This light or energy is the potency of the remedy and is unique to each making and each individual essence.'[6] Once the essence is made, the essence then holds this resonance. He explains, 'The flower essence becomes a vehicle for preserving and transferring this light resonance to another person in another place.'[7] In other words, once an essence is made, bottled and distributed, many can benefit from its qualities. Dr Fritz-Albert Popp (discussed in Chapter 1, 'Energy, What and Who You Are'), wrote the following. 'We know today that man, essentially, is a being of light'[8] I am particularly drawn to his following statement, 'For humans, there was another possibility. If we could take in the photons of other living things, we might also be able to use the information from them to correct our own light if it went awry.'[9] Vibrational essences do just this!

This light resonance or energy pattern is sustained because water has the ability to hold a memory. This theory was first explored by a French scientist, Jacques Benveniste (1935–2004), in 1998, who experimented with an antibody diluted in water.[10] This solution was further diluted until the chance that a single molecule of antibody being left was very small. However, tests for properties related to the presence of the antibody proved positive — the water had retained the memory. It may seem far-fetched that water can hold an energetic pattern in this way, but this has been demonstrated more recently by the experiments of the late Dr Masaru Emoto (1943–2014), a Japanese scientist. In his book, *Messages from Water*, he provides photographic evidence showing how human consciousness has an effect on the molecular structure of water.[11] His experiments focused on exposing water to spoken and written words and projected thoughts or emotions. After freezing this water, the ice crystals either formed into beautiful patterns or distorted, broken arrangements dependent on whether the words, thoughts and emotions were kind, loving and peaceful or angry, violent and aggressive.

In 2020, leading German scientists examined individual drops of water at an incredibly high magnification, this enabled them to see that each droplet of water has its own individual microscopic pattern, each distinguishable from the next and uniquely beautiful. A scientific experiment was carried out whereby a group of students were encouraged to obtain one drop of water from the same body of water, all at the same time. Through close examination of the individual droplets, it was seen that each produced a different image. A second experiment was then carried out where a real flower was placed into a body of water, and after a while a sample droplet of the water was taken out for examination. The result produced a mesmerizing pattern when hugely magnified, but all of the droplets of this water looked very similar. When the same experiment was done with a different species of flower, the magnified droplet looked completely different, thereby determining that the energetic form of a particular flower is evident in each droplet of water.[12] Experiments such as these, confirm how the energetic pattern of a flower can be preserved in water. Additionally, considering our bodies are composed of a high percentage of water, Dr Emoto's experiments add further validity as to the power our emotions, thoughts and intentions can have on our physical form. Of further interest in regard to crystals is that scientists recognise that the water in our bodies is of a liquid crystalline structure. Read more about this in Chapter 6, 'We Are Crystals'.

It is essential to remind ourselves constantly that the energetic nature of our thoughts and feelings have the ability to affect us physically; they (we) are instrumental in creating our reality. Emotions such as worry, envy, anger and resentment resonate to a low frequency and are definitely not in our best interests, for example, living with, fear or the inability to forgive can be toxic to our bodies. Mahatma Gandhi's (1869–1948) quote is both humbling yet inspiring, 'The weak can never forgive. Forgiveness is the attribute of the strong.'[13] When it comes to fear, and its tendency to be disabling on many fronts, Julia Cannon emphasises the importance of believing in one's own convictions. Julia, initially a nurse, has explored other aspects of the healing profession including training in Re-connective Healing and Dolores Cannon's Quantum Healing Hypnosis Therapy, and is also author of *Soul Speak — The Language of Your Body*. She writes, 'Fear is lack of trust: in oneself, those around us and the world at large. So maybe the lesson we are trying to teach ourselves is to trust. Trust the universe, but ultimately, trust ourselves. We have the best indicators for our messages and growth right in our core. It's just a matter of tapping in and listening and not being afraid to experience the emotion to see the message that is being delivered.'[14] A vibrational essence holds a high vibrational frequency, which when ingested, has the ability to resonate with negative feelings such as these above, ameliorating or totally dissolving them. This may not happen instantly because humans are complex creatures, often with deep-seated issues to be resolved, but over a period of time and successive treatments consisting of (probably) several different essences. A typical treatment can often involve identifying and addressing many different layers of emotional and psychological issues (for example, anxieties, feelings of guilt), although they may not all necessarily present themselves initially. It can be a process over a period of time, much like peeling the layers of an onion. Over the years we can become cluttered with destructive emotions and beliefs that obscure our genuine self, we lose awareness of who we are; our inner true self is hidden. The more layers that are peeled away and resolved enables the light of the soul and our true purpose in life to shine through. According to Richard Gerber M.D. (1954–2007), 'The concept that human beings are dynamic energy systems which reflect evolutionary patterns of soul growth is the main tenet underlying vibrational medicine.'[15] The length of treatment may also depend on how long an issue has existed and how deeply it is ingrained into one's psyche. The intention with vibrational essences is to always resolve the core of the problem, however deep.

It is not just memories, deeply held destructive emotions and thought patterns that can impress upon our physical health. When we experience a shock, physically or emotionally, even if it is not a lasting trauma, this can upset the arrangement of the subtle energy bodies, causing them to become out of alignment. Misalignment can mean they are too far apart from each other, or in the case they are too close, this may result in their properties spilling over and becoming inappropriately linked. This can result in all sorts of problems such as, fear, anxiety, panic attacks, confusion, and lack of concentration. Obviously, this is not very helpful as maintaining an appropriate space and harmonious balance between the subtle bodies is very important. Additionally, the life force will be unable to flow correctly, creating a debilitating situation and undermining well-being. It is desirable that past shocks are neutralised as best they can be, otherwise the repercussions can become the basis for potential problems in the future. Living with an overload of shock, the etheric body eventually becomes depleted and less effective at protecting the physical body, so weaknesses may develop. Fortunately, essences can help because it appears they align and balance the subtle anatomy. Although there is at present little research into this area, when Kirlian photography[16] is used to take photographs of a person before and after taking vibrational essences, an expert specialised in analysing the result will be able to observe differences in energy fields and the chakras. These differences can indicate that imbalances, held as dissonant energies in the subtle anatomy, are restored.

Vibrational essences are important both as a treatment and in a preventative sense in that they help alleviate emotional distress and/or mental disturbances, prior to them potentially escalating to the stage in which they crystallize in the subtle bodies and cause later problems. When issues are resolved at an early stage this is obviously easier to deal with than at a later date. For instance, sadness, loss and grief are associated with the lungs. This theory derives from Chinese medicine but is also observed by many complementary therapies. It is preferable to ameliorate these emotions as best they can be and in whichever way is appropriate. If left raw and unsupported, eventually their effects may be experienced physically such as a lung problem, even years after an actual event or onset of feelings. There are many books based on similar 'mind/body link' concepts, which correlate feelings and emotions to actual parts and organs of the body and potential illnesses.[17] For example, the fear or inability to express oneself over a period of time, is likely to affect the throat chakra, which may impact on the correct functioning of the associated areas of the body, neck, throat and thyroid. It can be helpful to explore similar mind/body relationships applicable to oneself so as to improve (perhaps through taking vibrational essences) dysfunctional patterns and re-establish a healthy relationship between one's mind and body.

One of the most helpful reasons for taking essences is that they gently awaken one as to what needs to change within oneself and assist one in seeing one's life experiences in a different way. They help to develop a greater understanding of who one is, so one becomes more conscious of what is in one's own best interests. Essences also help us become more familiar with a higher aspect of ourselves as Richard Gerber M.D. (1954–2007) explains. 'When we become more spiritually aware and in tune with the inner guidance of our Higher Selves, the mechanisms by which we can change our emotions, our minds, our bodies, and our lives, become more apparent. For instance, flower essences contain the very energies of pure consciousness that allow the connections between the lower and higher selves to be re-established.'[18] On this subject, Dr Bach writes, 'Disease is in essence the result of conflict between Soul and Mind, and will never be eradicated except by spiritual and mental effort.'[19] He continues, 'that so long as our Souls and personalities are in harmony all is joy and peace, happiness and health.'[20]

Dr Bach recognised that for illness to be healed, one should treat the actual person rather than their symptoms. This was also his ethos regarding how vibrational essences work and is observed by registered practitioners (www.bfvea.com or www.bachcentre.com) of flower essence therapy. In the UK, no claim that vibrational essences heal, or cure can be made as vibrational essences are not classified as medicines. Vibrational essences do not directly affect the physical form, but it is only after mental tribulations or problems of an emotional nature are resolved, that physical changes may transpire.[21] This premise is the underlying message of this book, to always address psychological imbalances as a priority. As an example, if after taking an essence to calm anxiety and worry, one may well find lessening of any uneasy knot feeling in the stomach, which typically accompanies worry and nervousness. Additionally, improvement of headaches may occur naturally after essences have decreased feelings of tension and strain. Vibrational essences are only the catalyst in this process; they transform one's mindset and the body often responds to this. Keeping in mind how the subtle anatomy works, Gurudas makes the point, 'flower essences adjust the flow of consciousness and karma that create the disease state. They influence the subtle bodies and ethereal properties of the anatomy, and then gradually influence the physical body.'[22] Gurudas expands on how essences influence the physical body, 'they merely create a clear state of consciousness, which then affects the personality, the physical body....' Although research into vibrational essences is very much in its infancy, it is observed by Kirlian photography that essences positively affect the subtle anatomy. Physical changes may therefore result due to the effect of an essence on a chakra and the chakra's connection with the endocrine system.

Once a chakra is rebalanced, it will perform more optimally. The physical body operates as a receiver, a physical malfunction is not the primary cause of illness and disease, although obviously we have to accept the ageing process. The subtle anatomy system must be healed/rebalanced (in whatever way appropriate) as a priority before any physical outcomes are noticed, but this is not guaranteed especially if it is not in the soul's remit to get better. In this case, essences can bring an awareness of the reasons behind an illness and/or provide acceptance and understanding of a current health situation that may previously had not been possible.

As a vibrational essence is a frequency it therefore has the power to transcend the limits of space and time (if indeed there is such a thing as time, according to quantum physics) when it comes to our past feelings. If the past involves unfavourable conditioning or memories of an unpleasant nature, essences help reframe these, enabling one to establish healthier patterns for the future. In this context, essences may also help with the psychological issues behind inherited miasms (written about in Chapter 9). Miasms hold memories of potential illnesses and disease patterns originating from past generations and once they enter the physical body, they are thought to become embodied in the DNA and can cause the breakdown of the body's immune defences. Homeopathic thinking is that if they can be dissolved, the body is brought back into wholeness and strength again. If a miasm is a latent ancestral energy, then the assumption must be that the psychological themes associated with it are also passed by predecessors as well as the physical predispositions. If our bodies are repositories of everything derived from our ancestral bloodline, one can only imagine the legacy of tremendous loss, abuse, trauma, sadness etc., that is passed through numerous generations. These energetic ties can keep us bound to our ancestors; past entanglements are intertwined with our ancestors' beliefs and behaviours, so there may not be a choice in taking on these suppressed psychological traits. Another perspective on this is that one may have chosen (a pre-birth decision) to work on issues that members in past generations, for whatever reasons, did not. It takes courage to be the 'cycle breaker', the one who refuses to further carry debilitating psychological burdens that incapacitate, and hamper living life to the full. Gurudas emphasises accountability when discussing inherited miasms, which he believes are more directly linked to the individual's consciousness. He explains the word 'inherited' implies that the physical body is somehow subjected to the planned ancestral lineage of an individual to find a karmic focus within their particular body. He writes, 'Inherited miasms and various diseases are reflective of many of the soul's activities. Thus, these imbalances are karmically originated as the soul expresses or activates itself in a physical body. The inherited miasms become a portal, particularly as they align with the chakras, through which other miasms become active expressions of either blockages or enhancers to the progression of the soul in its quest to obtain knowledge of itself as a spiritual being by placing itself under the discipline of the body physical.'[23]

It is crucial to be aware of and ensure one does not continue to hold onto unsupportive behavioural patterns thus energising destructive emotions and jeopardising health as a result. Our assumption in the past has been that we are destined to be controlled by our DNA, we are helpless to do anything about this, but through the science of Epigenetics, mentioned earlier in this book, we now know that this is no longer considered true. The main messages of Bruce Lipton's book reinforce what many in complementary therapies already believe, the importance of re-programming the mind, as it is our perceptions not our genes that control our biology.[24] Miasms cannot be cleared with traditional medicine as they are a vibrational problem. Gurudas alludes to vibrational essences helping to remove miasms: 'Flower essences do not so much directly abate the miasms; they merely create a clear state of consciousness, which then affects the personality, the physical body, and the genetic code and may entirely eliminate miasms from the physical body and subtle bodies.'[25] In his book,[26] Ian Watson, an advocate of using vibrational essences to clear miasms, includes suggestions of various flower essences which relate to the core psychological themes behind each miasm.

During his work in treating root causes of chronic problems (using psychotherapy and energy work), Tomislav Budak conducted independent research of miasms and discovered some interesting characteristics of their dynamics and anatomy. He advises the best way to dissolve a miasm is to use more than one approach. He writes, 'However, optimal results are achieved if consciousness (the brain and nervous system) is also involved in the healing process. Healing can be achieved much faster when it is simultaneously based on both correcting the life force and becoming aware of the causes of the problems, of the influence they have and, on their meaning, the lesson hidden behind it.'[27] He advocates forms of psychotherapy that work at a deep level. Another option is to use liquid psychotherapy, that is vibrational essences to reprogramme well-being, emotionally, mentally and spiritually. Vibrational essences have the ability to transform unhelpful emotions and thought patterns that have been inherited from past family members. This not only creates improved future patterns of health for oneself, but also for forthcoming generations. According to Ian Watson[28] miasms correspond to different chakras. As flower and gem essences are thought to work at the chakra and subtle body level, it seems logical to use them.

Vibrational essences appear to work by interacting with the subtle anatomy and enhancing the connection between higher aspects of our consciousness and our rational minds. Like humans, each plant and flower have a unique frequency, so when a vibrational essence is ingested, a specific frequency is delivered to our energetic multi-dimensional system. It is believed that after resonating with disturbed frequencies, a harmonic retuning takes place, bringing about a state of internal harmony in this system, and enhancing our life force. Naturally, this reflects positively on the physical and cellular patterns in the body, decreasing the opportunity for potential changes of a detrimental nature. In *Flower Essences and Vibrational Healing*, Gurudas explains, 'When there is a sympathetic bonding and it begins to act on the physical body, emotional tensions that get locked into the DNA even down to the molecular level cannot hold their presence and permeate the physical form.'[29]

He describes the process in that, after ingestion, vibrational essences are firstly assimilated into the circulatory system, settle midway between the nervous and circulatory systems and then go directly to the meridians. He references Alice Bailey to explain what happens to the nervous and circulatory systems, 'An electromagnetic current is created here by the polarity of these two systems. Indeed, there is an intimate connection between these two systems in relation to the life force and consciousness that modern science does not yet understand.'[30] To explain this further, it is worth repeating Gurudas' quote, 'The life force works more through the blood, and consciousness works more through the brain and nervous system. These two systems contain quartz-like properties and electromagnetic currents. The blood cells, especially the red and white blood cells, contain more quartz-like properties, and the nervous system contains more electromagnetic current. The life force and consciousness use these properties to enter and stimulate the physical body.'[31] It appears these quartz-like properties which form part of the crystalline system in the physical and subtle bodies (described in Chapter 6, 'We Are Crystals') augment the impact of vibrational essences. 'Crystalline structures work on sympathetic resonancy. There is an attunement between crystalline properties in the physical and subtle bodies, the ethers, and many vibrational remedies, notably flower essences and gems.'[32] Richard Gerber M.D. (1954–2007) offers his opinion as to how this process works, 'There appears to be an entire subtle energetic network throughout the body that utilizes these bio-crystalline structures. This crystalline network is involved with the assimilation and processing of the subtle energies of vibrational remedies.'[33] Dr Mae Wan Ho confirms his view, 'There is a dynamic, liquid crystalline continuum of connective tissues and extracellular matrix linking directly into the equally liquid crystalline interior of every single cell in the body. Liquid crystallinity gives organisms their characteristic flexibility, exquisite sensitivity and responsiveness, thus optimizing the rapid, noiseless intercommunication that enables the organism to function as a coherent, coordinated whole. In addition, the liquid crystalline continuum provides subtle electrical interconnections which are sensitive to changes in pressure and other physicochemical conditions; in other words, it is also able to register "tissue memory". Thus, the liquid crystalline continuum possesses all the qualities of a highly sensitive "body consciousness" that can respond to all forms of subtle energy medicines.'[34] It also seems that the crystalline components of water contained in the human body play an important part in how essences work.

Although vibrational essences are a growing therapy, they are still in their infancy, as as a mindset change is necessary, one that embraces the concept (not currently widely held) that emotions and beliefs can affect one's health. Their use also requires a sense of self-responsibility and an openness to self-healing, and it is even better (although not necessary) if one recognises, 'if I was instrumental in creating a condition, then I can remove it.' Without an appreciation of energy, and because it works in an ethereal way currently at odds with traditional methods of treatment, medical circles are not familiar with the huge potential of a modality such as this. Alice Bailey's thoughts on this are, 'The centre of attention of medical and scientific students will be focused on the etheric body, and the dependence of the physical body upon the etheric body will be recognized. This will change the attitude of the medical profession, and magnetic healing and vibratory stimulation will supersede the present methods of surgery and drug assimilation.'[35]

Vibrational essences are used not just for therapeutic reasons but for personal development. Their use can facilitate a journey of self-discovery, promote inner growth, and raise spiritual awareness. Dr Bach believed that essences put us in touch with our higher selves. 'The action of these remedies is to raise our vibrations and open up our channels for the reception of our Spiritual Self....'[36]

In the final chapter, I focus on the importance of light to the physical body.

If we could see the miracle of a single flower clearly our whole life would change. **Buddha**[37]

Endnotes

1. Einstein quote. Available at https://quotefancy.com/ quote/762846/Albert-Einstein-Future-medicine-will-be-the-medicine-of-frequencies (Accessed: September 2022)

2. The Royal Rife Machine. *A Brief History of Dr. Royal Raymond Rife*. Available at https://www.royal-rife-machine.com/ Royal-Rife.htm (Accessed: October 2022)

3. Tesla's medicine. *The healing fields of Nikola Tesla*. Available at https://teslasmedicine.com/the-history-of-tesla-medicine/ (Accessed: November 2022)

4. Solfeggio frequencies. Available at https://www. naturehealingsociety.com/articles/solfeggio/ (Accessed: September 2022)

5. Barnard, J. (2002) *Bach Flower Remedies: Form and Function.* UK: Flower Remedy Programme, p. 68

6. Barnard, J. (2002) *Bach Flower Remedies: Form and Function.* UK: Flower Remedy Programme, p. 68

7. Barnard, J. (2002) *Bach Flower Remedies: Form and Function.* UK: Flower Remedy Programme, p. 244

8. Biophotonservices. *Dr Fritz Albert Popp.* Available at http://www.biophotonservices.com/dr-fritz-albert-popp/ (Accessed: September 2022)

9. Biontologyarizona. *Dr Fritz Albert Popp*. Available at http:// www.biontologyarizona.com/fritz-albert-popp-cure-for-cancer/ (Accessed: September 2022)

10. McTaggart, L. (2003) *The Field.* UK: Harper Collins Ltd

11. Emoto, M. (1999) *Messages from Water.* Tokyo: Hado Publishing

12. Resonance Science Foundation. *Scientists show that water has a memory.* Available at http://www.resonancescience.

org/blog/Scientists-Show-That%20Water-Has-Memory? fbclid=IwAR19JBotCKobSCLK6Isrf5znV76YW9ZXAl34eQf 6PY7AhSBOmIfwThD95CI (Accessed: September 2022)

13   Mahatma Gandhi quote. Available at http://www. goodreads.com/quotes/11741-the-weak-can-never-forgive-forgiveness-is-the-attribute-of (Accessed: September 2022)

14.   Cannon, J. (2013) *Soul Speak — The Language of Your Body.* Arkansas: Ozark Mountain Publishing, Chapter 5, p.26

15.   Gerber, R. (1996) V*ibrational Medicine. New Mexico:* Bear & Company Publishing, p. 468

16   Read about this photographic technology in Chapter 10.

17.   Segal, I. (2010) *Secret language of your Body: The Essential Guide to Health & Wellness.* USA: Beyond Words Publishing

18.   Gerber, R. (1996) V*ibrational Medicine. New Mexico:* Bear & Company Publishing, p. 487

19.   Bach, E. *Heal Thyself.* Available at https://www. bachflowerlearning.com/books/heal-thyself-ebook-version/ p. 7 (Accessed: September 2022)

20.   Bach, E. *Heal Thyself.* Available at https://www. bachflowerlearning.com/books/heal-thyself-ebook-version/ p. 11 (Accessed: September 2022)

21.   Essences should never be used as a substitute to seeking medical advice.

22.   Gurudas. (1986) *Gem Elixirs and Vibrational Healing, Vol. II.* California: One 70 Press, p.102

23.   Gurudas. (1986) *Gem Elixirs and Vibrational Healing, Vol. II.* California: One 70 Press, p.105

24.   Lipton, B. H. (2005) *The Biology of Belief.* UK: Cygnus Books

25.   Gurudas. (1986) *Gem Elixirs and Vibrational Healing, Vol. II.* California: One 70 Press, p. 102

26.   Watson, I. (2009) *The Homeopathic Miasms: A Modern View.* UK: Cutting Edge Publications

27.   Budak, T. *MIASMS — A New Perspective on the Hereditary Factor*

Available at http://www.tomislavbudak.com/en/articles/advanced/140-miasms-a-new-pespective (Accessed: September 2022)

28. Watson, I. (2009) *The Homeopathic Miasms: A Modern View.* UK: Cutting Edge Publications

29. Gurudas. (1986) *Gem Elixirs and Vibrational Healing, Vol. II.* California: One 70 Press, p.146

30. Gurudas. (1989) *Flower Essences and Vibrational Healing.* California: Cassandra Press, p. 27

31. Gurudas. (1989) *Flower Essences and Vibrational Healing.* California: Cassandra Press, p. 27

32. Gurudas. (1989) *Flower Essences and Vibrational Healing.* California: Cassandra Press, p. 28

33. Gerber, R. (1996) V*ibrational Medicine. New Mexico:* Bear & Company Publishing, p. 253

34. Ho, M.W. *Coherent Energy, Liquid Crystallinity and Acupuncture.* A talk presented to British Acupuncture Society, 2 October 1999, Available at https://www.i-sis.org.uk/acupunc.php (Accessed: September 2022)

35. Bailey, A. *A Treatise on Cosmic Fire.* London: Lucis Press, Limited, p. 474

36. Bach, E. *Ye Suffer from Yourselves.* This text was originally printed as a sixteen-page booklet and the contents given as a talk by Dr Edward Bach to a homeopathic society in Stockport, Lancashire in February 1931. Available from https://bachcentre.com/wp-content/uploads/2019/10/ye_suffer_from_yourselves_en.pdf p. 15. (Accessed: October 2022)

37. Buddha quote. Available at http://www.goodreads.com/quotes/56975-if-we-could-see-the-miracle-of-a-single-flower (Accessed: September 2022)

Chapter 12

It's All About Light

Nothing can dim the light which shines from within.
Maya Angelou[1]

In previous chapters I have described the subtle energy system and highlighted the importance of appreciating and managing ourselves as energy beings, especially in relation to our health. One vital theme of this book is that of 'light'. For instance, Prana fills the body with light, which is subsequently transformed into life force energy, we consist of slowed down sound and light waves and emit frequencies of light. Our whole metabolism depends on the function of light and particles of light transmit information within and between our cells. To change the frequency of an emotion or feeling, we need to change the quality of the light patterns that make up that reality, and one of the ways this can be achieved is through the use of vibrational treatments. Vibrational essences contain the light resonance or energy pattern of a flower or other physical sources or locations, which is sustained because water has the ability to hold a memory. This light memory, held in the essence, appears to correct our own light when it becomes misaligned. Light is not only crucial to our well-being, but in this final chapter, I explain how increasing fields of light are driving our growth and greater potential for well-being.

We are at a pivotal point in history where we are being affected by an evolutionary process which is causing the frequencies of our minds to accelerate and our bodies to change. The human energy field is being rewired to carry new energies and subsequently our bodies are readjusting accordingly. Although this process has been in progress for some years, it is accelerating, and currently we are experiencing a high growth spurt in our evolution. This will, ultimately, support an easier alignment with higher dimensions, and empower us to embrace our higher abilities and operate more fully as our true selves. Barbara Marciniak writes, 'On a subatomic level, your body is being deeply affected by the energies emanating from a vast array of celestial influences that are providing information in the form of light-encoded frequencies.'[2]

Barbara describes that at any point in time, the dimension that the majority of people experience defines the overall dimension of earth, and it appears this is an instinctive consensus. 'Humanity creates the world at large by way of unconscious primal mass agreements. You are participating in a mass agreement that is exploring the nature of reality from a 3-D vista,...'[3] It seems recently, however, that increasing light frequencies are reprogramming our brains to enable access to a much wider range of information than is currently available in the third dimension. Many people are awakening to the reality that as humans we extend beyond what is a solely third dimensional experience; we already have the (subtle) equipment to be conscious in other dimensions. Some people are realising that everything is frequency, and they (as a frequency) have the ability to choose how to perceive their reality from a higher dimensional perspective. As stated previously, this is especially helpful when undesirable things happen, as applying a higher viewpoint to situations and feelings can provide improved opportunities for how we approach and live our lives and what we establish in the future.

To return to the subject of light, most people are accustomed to thinking of light as something perceptible, but we know from the experiments of Dr Fritz Popp, we contain light internally. We can increase light within (and on a subtle level) by visualising it. Author Sanyana Roman (1949–2021), provides an understanding on how this can be done, 'If I were to say to you, "Connect with the light," you would instinctively know how to do that, for your Higher Self is always connected with light. As you think of light you begin to vibrate with your Higher Self. You can bring more light into your life by thinking of it. Light responds to your thoughts of it; as you think of it, it is immediately drawn to you. As you think of light more often you will become charged with light, building a radiant body of light all around you. The more light your body can hold, the higher your vibration and the greater your ability to transform the energy around you into a higher order.'[4] Dr Joshua Stone (1953–2005), influential spiritual teacher and author of several books on spiritual psychology, advocated anchoring greater and greater frequencies of light into each of our cells by using intention and desire. He uses the words 'light quotient' as a measurement of this and reminds us that at every moment of the day we are either building or decreasing our light quotient dependent on our thoughts, words and actions. He underlines the importance of stabilising the light as (not surprisingly), it can fluctuate according to what is going on in one's consciousness and life.[5]

As a result of what is happening in space/ethers, we are taking in higher frequencies of light. Beatriz Singer writes, 'Shifting frequencies means being able to encode more light, being in balance with the implicate and explicate[6] order within us, and seeing ourselves as not only separated individuals but also entangled parts of the whole and co-creators of a new authentic reality.'[7] All life is vibration, every form of matter is light and according to the vibration, the light goes into or exposes form. Vibration is light, we are light beings, just as everything else in creation, the difference being the frequency of light carried. It helps to have more conscious awareness of light generally and especially in visualising the light within. According to Dr Fritz Popp's experiments, light is within every cell of our bodies, we are shining with light. He believed that healing is a matter of reprogramming discordant light fluctuations, so they operate more coherently. Light carries information, light cannot hold illness, so it is most important we don't let our light go out. When the body holds higher frequencies, it starts to hold more light which is helped by its crystalline nature. Barbara Marciniak remarks, 'Light is electromagnetic radiation that travels in wave form, and your cells, which are crystalline in structure, eagerly respond to natural light.'[8] Barbara Wren a naturopath, nutritionist, healer and teacher, has over many years, investigated how our bodies hold and create light. In her book she explains the body's potential to receive and transmit the full spectrum of light. 'Light not only comes in from the universe but is also produced by free radicals coming together at great speed. This internally-produced light is referred to as bio-photons. Our DNA personalizes the light from the universe. It holds the imprint of who we are, and when we are fully functioning and able to make and emit bio-photons, we are able to fully manifest who we are.'[9]

When we consciously raise our light level by cultivating calm, living in joy, being in nature and thinking good of others, we increase our vibration, and our light levels are amplified to an extent where lower frequency emotions are unable to exist. This makes it much harder to hold onto unnecessary emotional baggage or dysfunctional beliefs, which we often erroneously believe define who we are. In these challenging times, we are being pushed to purge what is no longer a part of who we need to be in order to survive with peace of mind in the future and reach our highest potential. When our vibration lightens, the tendency is for our unresolved 'stuff' to surface for resolution, whether we want it to or not! Uncomfortable as it may be, it is in our best interest to let go of or rewrite those elements in the past that have an emotional hold over us. When we do this, our vibration reflects this and circumstances are then drawn towards us that match our higher vibration, placing us in a more advantageous position to create and experience a positive future. Our subconscious mind does not know the difference between what we feel about the past or what we feel now, that is why it is important to cultivate mastery over our thoughts and feelings, so we can dictate how we want to feel. To take that mastery of thoughts a step further and keeping in mind that cell regeneration is a biological feature of all living organisms, it is advisable to reaffirm our cells regenerate perfectly. To avoid a new cell automatically copying a damaged cell (such as in disease or illness), it is essential to use our thoughts to instruct our cells to regenerate in perfect balance and wholeness, otherwise we may risk it renewing defectively. Above all, emotional stability and clear thinking must be our priority in the next stage of our journey and when we live constantly in the heart we feed our cells with happiness, love, joy and peace, and we know our cells are listening!

Light can be thought of as wisdom and spiritual consciousness (as mentioned in Chapter 6 'The Seven Rays of Light'). There are certain times, in the process of humanity's evolution, such as now, when a fresh release of spiritual illumination is discharged to the earth plane which triggers transformative events in the world. This could be ascribable to many different factors, the energies of the Seventh Ray, the Aquarian Age and the convergence and culmination of several cosmic cycles which have taken place in recent years. Additionally, there is a belief, that Earth has in recent years, moved into a highly charged region of space near the Pleiades, called the Photon Belt[10] (also referred to as Photon Band, Photon Ring or Golden Nebula), said to be discovered by astronauts in 1961 by means of satellite-borne instruments. It is thought our solar system enters this area of the galaxy every 11,000 years for a period of 2,000 years in its 26,000-year orbit of the galactic centre, the centre of the Milky Way Galaxy. Although much is written about this belt and its effects on humanity, there is little published science to support it. However, Nasa's claim in 2009,[11] that the solar system was passing through an interstellar cloud that physics say should not exist, is thought, by many, to be evidence of the Photon Belt. The last time this happened was during the time of Atlantis, and it is believed, as was then, it will usher in a 'Golden Age'.

It appears that as we travel through new areas of space, we are exposed to energy transmissions that alter our physicality and the framework of our existing reality. Susan Joy Rennison, who has an honours degree in physics and geophysics and works as an independent researcher, suggested in 2006[12] that another contributing factor to transformative world events is that we are experiencing space weather[13] which is a result of the changing conditions in space. The author speculates whether space weather is a consequence of our position in the Photon Belt. She explains that space weather is now a fact of life and is causing us to evolve. 'Space weather is a consequence of the behaviour of the Sun, the nature of Earth's magnetic field and atmosphere, and our location in the solar system. The active elements of space weather are particles, electromagnetic energy and magnetic fields, rather than the more commonly known weather contributors of water, temperature and air. Magnetic fields, radiation, particles and matter which have been ejected from the Sun can interact with the Earth's magnetic field and upper atmosphere to produce a variety of effects.'[14] Certainly, in recent years, we had seen radical weather patterns, earth changes and there has been unprecedented solar activity, perhaps an indication that the consciousness of our solar system is itself also undergoing an upgrade in frequency (read Chapter 4, 'We Are All One'). In a similar vein, and especially pertinent to our health, many readers may be familiar with fluctuations of the Schumann resonance.[15]

Due to our increasing awareness, it now seems incredulous to many that for thousands of years humanity has been kept distracted from knowing their true selves and spiritual identities. They have been kept diverted from being able to utilise their own power for the benefit of their health or to create a better world. Many people are now peering out of what appears to be a matrix in which we have been imprisoned and disempowered, only to discover who we really are and that we have the skills to become conscious creators of our lives. This is a typical manifestation of the lower energies of Sixth Ray and Age of Pisces. As their power fades, greater knowledge of hidden agendas, nefarious manipulation and deception is coming to the surface and into the light to be removed. As we are evolving, we are moving beyond collective conscious belief patterns that have programmed and enslaved us for many years, we are waking up from an illusion. For example, we have been conditioned to believe in a narrative that affirms we should trust in the external, whether that is someone in authority, or a belief system. As we break away from these limiting beliefs, we are learning to trust in ourselves, our feelings and intuitions and to resonate with higher knowledge.

One tool helping humanity to purify their physical and energy bodies and cleanse illusions from their minds is the diamond consciousness, which brings transparency in enabling the truth to be seen. The quality of the energies (from the cosmos) now experienced is referred to in many circles as diamond light, or diamond consciousness. It is interesting to note that Penney Peirce refers to the soul as diamond light (read about the soul in Chapter 2) as the diamond is said to be an important shape that enables us to receive higher energies. Susan Joy Rennison writes extensively in her book about the diamond shape formation apparent in galaxies, and that the earth's core is actually a diamond. Referring to its presence in the energy field, she writes, 'The "layers upon layers of light and energy" is the explanation for the emergence of the diamond, as there are refraction points associated with each layer.'[16] Her research uncovered that, 'The existence of diamond shape energetic structures in our energy fields was part of the "underground stream" of knowledge held in esoteric organizations and passed on to initiates.'[17] She continues, 'The diamond geometry is the perfect receiver and transmitter of electromagnetic signals, thus in this time of electromagnetic chaos, it is imperative that we only pick up the most beneficial electromagnetic signals to recode our DNA. So, as our DNA alters rapidly, we now have the energetic tools to help us radically transmute ourselves at the subatomic level and fully embody our divine and multidimensional nature.'[18]

We know from space weather that our planet is being showered with high frequency cosmic rays and the natural protective shields are weakening; it is a scientific fact. Not surprisingly our energy fields are changing to accommodate these new energies which are essentially heightening our levels of consciousness. Julie Umpleby, teacher, energy worker and healer-therapist, believes this change is bringing a greater (higher) level of order or coherence to our auric field enabling us to move forward through further energetic shifts whilst holding a stable and balanced core of higher energy. She considers that the diamond (or octahedron[19]) is an energy tool for maintaining balance during the challenging times in which we live, and it acts as an energy 'container' for the increased frequencies that both we and our planet are experiencing. 'The greater coherence is brought about through development and anchoring of an actual diamond grid of light in our energy field. This diamond grid of light facilitates the transmission of tremendous spiritual and healing power or energy. These individual diamonds ultimately link up forming a network or grid of diamond light around the planet.... The diamond is part of our current evolutionary process, and will help us to adjust to holding the greater electrical "charge" of our divine essence.'[20] Further confirmation of the significance of diamond energy may arise as the Seventh Ray increases in power, as this

Ray is connected not only to the mineral kingdom (crystals) but sacred geometry.

Many people may believe our current health system is not always making us better or keeping us healthy, financial conflicts may be the source of this. Neither is it designed to take into consideration that we are multidimensional energy light beings. Fortunately, we have more power than we think over our well-being and in our ability to maintain health. As we have seen throughout this book, we are certainly more than meets the eye, considerably more than most of us could ever imagine. I outline how we can take matters into our own hands by utilising our personal 'mind medicine' toolkit. Read the sections on the Emotional and Mental bodies in Chapter 2, 'The Subtle Anatomy — The Esoteric Constitution of a Human' — The Etheric Body. Developing proficiency in the skill of creating affirmative, constructive thoughts enables one to positively influence well-being and, working at this level may decrease the likelihood of health deteriorating or ill health establishing in the first place. Understanding ourselves from an energetic perspective is imperative and will ultimately lead to the transformation of the existing medical system where current interventions will ultimately be replaced by treatments that work at an energetic level. This means us; we are our own energetic treatment. In the future, living will depend to a greater extent on our ability to manage our multidimensional energetic self, embrace our innate intuitive faculties and higher wisdom and raise our light vibration. Are you up for the task?

May the light be with you. Shine on beautiful souls!

Imagining yourself to be the body,
no wonder you have all these ailments.
Imagining yourself to be the mind,
no wonder you have all these worries.

Knowing yourself to be consciousness,
no wonder there is all this space and peace.
Realising you are the unborn awareness,
no wonder you are supremely happy. **Mooji**[21]

Endnotes

1. Maya Angelou quote. Available at https://www.goodreads. com/quotes/67751-nothing-can-dim-the-light-which-shines-from-within (Accessed: September 2022)

2. From the book *Path of Empowerment.* Copyright © 2004 by Barbara Marciniak, p.135 Reprinted with permission by New World Library, Novato, CA. www.newworldlibrary.com

3. From the book *Path of Empowerment.* Copyright © 2004 by Barbara Marciniak, p.93 Reprinted with permission by New World Library, Novato, CA. www.newworldlibrary.com

4. Roman, Sanaya (1989) *Spiritual Growth: Being Your Higher Self.* p. 19. Information at www.orindaben.com. Excerpted with permission. Printed form published by H J Kramer a division of New World Library

5. Stone, J. David. (1995) *Beyond Ascension.* Arizona: Light Technology Publishing, LLC

6. Bladon, L. The Two sides of Reality. Implicate order and explicate order were coined by Nobel winning theoretical physicist David Bohm, and are used to describe two different frameworks for understanding the same phenomenon or aspect of reality. The Explicate Order is what we commonly refer to as reality, but this is actually only the external surface of reality. It is the familiar manifest world of space, time and matter. The Implicate Order is the deeper, more fundamental reality that underlies the familiar material surface. It is the unmanifest potentiality from which the manifest universe originates and emerges into actuality. Available at https://evolvingsouls.com/blog/two-sides-of-reality/ (Accessed: September 2022)

7. Singer, B. (2019) *The Crystal Blueprint*. UK: Hay House, p. 257

8. From the book *Path of Empowerment*. Copyright © 2004 by Barbara Marciniak, p.45 Reprinted with permission by New World Library, Novato, CA. www.newworldlibrary. com

9. Wren, B. (2009) *Cellular Awakening*. UK: Hay House, p. 54

10. Photon Belt Phenomenon. Available at https://www. youtube.com/watch?v=n9JdSTT2p24 See also De Villiers, Dr Y. Entering the Void: Episode 2 - The Photon Belt Available at https://www.youtube.com/watch?v=53v7ao2 i36U&t=705s (Accessed: September 2022)

11. NASA Science. (2009) *Voyager Makes an Interstellar Discovery*. Available at https://science.nasa.gov/science-news/science-at-nasa/2009/23dec_voyager (Accessed: September 2022)

12. Rennison, S. J. (2008) *Tuning the Diamonds: Electromagnetism & Spiritual Evolution*. 2nd edition. England: Joyfire Publishing

13. Razam, R. (2011) *Space weather: A talk with Susan Joy Rennison*. Available at https://realitysandwich.com/space_weather_talk_susan_joy_rennison/ (Accessed: September 2022)

14. What Is Space Weather. Available at https://www.metoffice. gov.uk/weather/learn-about/space-weather/what-is-space-weather (Accessed: September 2022)

15. Schumann resonance. Available at https://noc.galacticage. org/schumann-resonance/ (Accessed: September 2022)

16. Rennison, S. J. (2008) *Tuning the Diamonds: Electromagnetism & Spiritual Evolution*. 2nd edition. England: Joyfire Publishing, p. 255

17. Rennison, S. J. (2008) *Tuning the Diamonds: Electromagnetism & Spiritual Evolution*. 2nd edition. England: Joyfire Publishing, p. 192

18. Rennison, S. J. (2008) *Tuning the Diamonds: Electromagnetism & Spiritual Evolution.* 2nd edition. England: Joyfire Publishing, p. 192

19. The terms diamond and octahedron refer to the same thing.

20. Umpleby, J. *The Diamonds in Your Energy Field.* Available at https://www.diamondlightworld.net/article-diamonds.html (Accessed: September 2022)

21. Mooji, from *White Fire: Spiritual Insights and Teachings of Advaita Zen Master Mooji* (2020). UK: Mooji Media Publications Limited, p. 111

About the Author

Debbie Sellwood brings to this book years of experience of working with energy. After a career in IT, she has for more than the last 20 years, worked as an advanced Flower Essence practitioner (bfvea.com). This modality recognises that humans comprise of a complex spectrum of electromagnetic energy frequencies which are related to our emotions and thinking. When vibrational essences are taken, out of balance emotions or negative thoughts are transmuted resulting in bringing equilibrium to the human condition.

For most of her adult life she has been interested in natural ways of healing and using the force of consciousness as a tool for empowerment, emotionally, mentally and in a health sense. As long as she can remember she has had an interest in how people tick, which led her to become a professional Astrologer (www.professionalastrologers.co.uk). She is passionate about helping people understand who they really are so they can become their true authentic selves and make decisions that are in their best interests.

Debbie lives in Hampshire, UK, with her husband. She is the mother of three grown up children and seven grandchildren. She has an interest in metaphysics and ancient mysteries and enjoys sewing, gardening and being in nature.

www.debbiesellwood.com

Bibliography

Bailey, A. A. (2005) *A Treatise on Cosmic Fire*. London: Lucis Press, Limited

Bailey, A. A. (2014) *A Treatise on White Magic*. London: Lucis Press, Limited

Bailey, A. A. (2007) *Esoteric Healing*. London: Lucis Press, Limited

Bailey, A. A. (2003) *The Seven Rays of Life*. London: Lucis Press, Limited

Barnard, J. (2002) *Bach Flower Remedies: Form and Function*. UK: Flower Remedy Programme

Barrett, S. (2013) *Secrets of your Cells*. Colorado: Sounds True, Inc

Bartlett, R. (2009) *The Physics of Miracles*. New York: Atria Books

Bentov, I. (1998) *Stalking the Wild Pendulum*. USA: Inner Traditions

Bohm, D. (2002) *Wholeness and the Implicate Order*. UK: Routledge

Brennan, B. A. (1988) *Hands of Light*. New York: Bantam Books

Brennan, B. A. (1993) *Light Emerging*. New York: Bantam Books

Burr, H. S. (1972) *The Fields of Life: Our links with the Universe*. New York: Ballantine Books

Cannon, J. (2013) *Soul Speak: The language of your body*. Arkansas: Ozark Mountain Publishing

Cousens, G. (2005) *Spiritual Nutrition: Six Foundations for Spiritual Life*. USA: North Atlantic Books

Currivan, J. (2017) *The Cosmic Hologram*. USA: Inner Traditions

Emoto, M. (1999) *Messages from Water*. Tokyo: Hado Publishing

Gerber, R. (1996) *Vibrational Medicine*. New Mexico: Bear & Company Publishing

Glasson, N. S. (2010) *The Twelve Rays of Light*. UK: Derwen Publishing

Griscom, C. (1986) *Time is an Illusion*. USA: Simon Schuster

Gurudas. (1989) *Flower Essences and Vibrational Healing.* California: Cassandra Press Gurudas. (1985) *Gem Elixirs and Vibrational Healing, Vol. I.* California: Cassandra Press

Gurudas. (1986) *Gem Elixirs and Vibrational Healing, Vol. II.* California: One 70 Press

Hall, J. (2003) *The Crystal Bible,* UK: Godsfield Press

Hawkins, D. (2014) *Power vs. Force: The Hidden Determinants of Human Behaviour.* UK: Hay House

Ho, MW. (2008) *The Rainbow and the Worm: The Physics of Organisms.* Singapore: World Scientific Publishing Company

Hodgson, J. (1986) *Why on Earth.* England: The White Eagle Publishing Trust

Hodgson, J. (1985) *Astrology: The Sacred Science.* England: The White Eagle Publishing Trust

Hunt, V. (1996) *Infinite Mind: Science of the Human Vibrations of Consciousness.* USA: Malibu Publishers

Laszlo, E. (1995) *Interconnected Universe: Conceptual Foundations of Transdisciplinary Unified Theory.* Singapore: World Scientific

Lipton, B. H. (2005) *The Biology of Belief.* UK: Cygnus Books

Marciniak, B. *Path of Empowerment.* Copyright © 2004, Reprinted with permission by New World Library, Novato, CA. www. newworldlibrary.com

McTaggart, L. (2003) *The Field.* UK: Harper Collins Ltd

McTaggart, L. (2017) *The Power of Eight.* UK: Hay House

Meader, W. A. (2004) *Shine Forth: The Soul's Magical Destiny.* California: Source Publications

Mooji, (2020) *White Fire: Spiritual Insights and Teachings of Advaita Zen Master Mooji.* UK: Mooji Media Publications Limited. All quotes by Mooji are (c) Mooji Media Ltd, www.mooji.org

Mossop, D. (1997) *The Power of Plants.* Jersey, UK: The Institute of Phytobiophysics

Myss, C. (1997) *Anatomy of the Spirit.* New York: Bantam

Oschman, J. L. (2000) *Energy Medicine: The Scientific Basis.* California: Harcourt Publishers Ltd

Pangman, M. J and Evans, M. (2017) *Dancing with Water.* 2nd edition. USA: Uplifting Press

Peirce, P. (2009) *Frequency.* New York: Atria Books

Pert, C. (1998) *Molecules of Emotion.* London: Simon & Schuster UK Ltd

Pollack, G. (2001) *Cells, Gels & the Engines of Life: A New Unifying Approach to Cell Function.* USA: Ebner and Sons Publishers

Pollack, G. (2013) *The Fourth Phase of Water.* USA: Ebner and Sons Publishers

Rennison, S. J. (2008 2nd edition) *Tuning the Diamonds: Electromagnetism & Spiritual Evolution.* England: Joyfire Publishing

Reyner, J. H, in collaboration with Laurence, G, and Upton, C. (2001) *Psionic Medicine.* UK: The C.W. Daniel Company Limited

Roman, S. (1989) *Spiritual Growth: Being your Higher Self.* California: Printed form published by H J Kramer a division of New World Library

Segal, I. (2010) *Secret language of your Body: The Essential Guide to Health & Wellness.* USA: Beyond Words Publishing

Singer, B. (2019) *The Crystal Blueprint*, UK: Hay House

Stephenson, M. (2008) *The Sage Age.* USA: Nightengale Press

Stone, J. D. (1995) *Beyond Ascension.* Arizona: Light Technology Publishing, LLC

Talbot, M. (1991) *The Holographic Universe.* New York: Harper Collins Publishers

Tolle, E. (2001) *The Power of Now.* UK: Hodder and Stoughton

Vywamus. (Channelled by Janet McClure) (1989) *Scopes of Dimensions.* Arizona: 3 Light Technology Publishing

Watson, I. (2009) *The Homeopathic Miasms: A Modern View.* UK: Cutting Edge Publications

Wren, B. (2009) *Cellular Awakening.* UK: Hay House

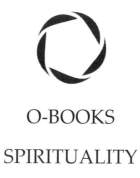

O-BOOKS

SPIRITUALITY

O is a symbol of the world, of oneness and unity; this eye
represents knowledge and insight. We publish titles on general
spirituality and living a spiritual life. We aim to inform and
help you on your own journey in this life.
If you have enjoyed this book, why not tell other readers
by posting a review on your preferred book site?

Recent bestsellers from O-Books are:

Heart of Tantric Sex
Diana Richardson
Revealing Eastern secrets of deep love and intimacy
to Western couples.
Paperback: 978-1-90381-637-0 ebook: 978-1-84694-637-0

Crystal Prescriptions
The A-Z guide to over 1,200 symptoms and their healing crystals
Judy Hall
The first in the popular series of eight books, this handy little
guide is packed as tight as a pill bottle with crystal remedies
for ailments.
Paperback: 978-1-90504-740-6 ebook: 978-1-84694-629-5

Shine On

David Ditchfield and J S Jones

What if the aftereffects of a near-death experience were undeniable? What if a person could suddenly produce high-quality paintings of the afterlife, or if they acquired the ability to compose classical symphonies? Meet: David Ditchfield.

Paperback: 978-1-78904-365-5 ebook: 978-1-78904-366-2

The Way of Reiki

The Inner Teachings of Mikao Usui

Frans Stiene

The roadmap for deepening your understanding of the system of Reiki and rediscovering your True Self.

Paperback: 978-1-78535-665-0 ebook: 978-1-78535-744-2

You Are Not Your Thoughts.

Frances Trussell

The journey to a mindful way of being, for those who want to truly know the power of mindfulness.

Paperback: 978-1-78535-816-6 ebook: 978-1-78535-817-3

The Mysteries of the Twelfth Astrological House

Fallen Angels

Carmen Turner-Schott, MSW, LISW

Everyone wants to know more about the most misunderstood house in astrology — the twelfth astrological house.

Paperback: 978-1-78099-343-0 ebook: 978-1-78099-344-7

WhatsApps from Heaven
Louise Hamlin
An account of a bereavement and the extraordinary
signs — including WhatsApps — that a retired
law lecturer received from her deceased husband.
Paperback: 978-1-78904-947-3 ebook: 978-1-78904-948-0

The Holistic Guide to Your Health
& Wellbeing Today
Oliver Rolfe
A holistic guide to improving your complete health,
both inside and out.
Paperback: 978-1-78535-392-5 ebook: 978-1-78535-393-2

Cool Sex
Diana Richardson and Wendy Doeleman
For deeply satisfying sex, the real secret is to reduce the heat,
to cool down. Discover the empowerment and fulfilment
of sex with loving mindfulness.
Paperback: 978-1-78904-351-8 ebook: 978-1-78904-352-5

Creating Real Happiness A to Z
Stephani Grace
Creating Real Happiness A to Z will help you understand
the truth that you are not your ego
(conditioned self).
Paperback: 978-1-78904-951-0 ebook: 978-1-78904-952-7

A Colourful Dose of Optimism
Jules Standish
It's time for us to look on the bright side, by boosting
our mood and lifting our spirit, both in our interiors,
as well as in our closet.
Paperback: 978-1-78904-927-5 ebook: 978-1-78904-928-2

Readers of ebooks can buy or view any of these bestsellers by
clicking on the live link in the title. Most titles are published
in paperback and as an ebook. Paperbacks are available in
traditional bookshops. Both print and ebook formats are
available online.

Find more titles and sign up to our readers' newsletter at
www.o-books.com

Follow O books on Facebook at **O-books**

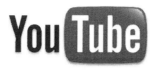

For video content, author interviews and more, please subscribe to our YouTube channel:

O-BOOKS Presents

Follow us on social media for book news, promotions and more:

Facebook: O-Books

Instagram: @o_books_mbs

Twitter: @obooks

Tik Tok: @ObooksMBS

www.o-books.com